38 WAYS TO DEVELOP YOUR BUST

BY

TED GAMBORDELLA

DEVELOPING THE RIGHT BUST DEVELOPMENT PROGRAM:
HOW TO USE THIS BOOK

Go through the entire book and do each exercise in the book at least twice for the first few After that, go back through the book and decide which exercises are most effective and enjoyable for your personality.

For maximun results, a personal exercise program should include:

★ 2 floor exercises
★ 1 "fly" or butterfly type exercise
★ 1 "decline" exercise, an exercise performed with the head lower than the feet
★ 1 incline exercise
★ 1 bench press, or flat bench
★ 1 "stretch" or full extension exercise

Once the exercise program is set, continue to do the selected exercises each day, or at least every other day, until the desired firmness and size is reached. Measure the bust, breast and chest area before beginning the program and decide on a goal immediately then keep up the program until that goal is reached.

If all the equipment called for is not available at home, join a spa. However, there are a number of exercises in this program which can be done without any equipment other than a few chairs, a towel and a wall. Exercises which call for an "incline board", for instance can be done using a slanted overturned lawn chair, or even off the edge of the bed. The photos and instructions contained in the exercise section of the book will suggest "at home" substitutions for the studio equipment found in health spas.

The most important thing is to get started on the exercises and continue to do them until the results are achieved. Most women can expect to feel and see some results in as little as a week, and can expect permanent results in only three months.

TABLE OF CONTENTS

FOREWARD

Since ancient times women have tried various potions and concoctions to help them to increase the size of their busts. A medieval alchemy book recommended tinture of arsenic, powdered lead, and rosewater...this to to mixed at midnight and spread on the breasts of a young virgin daily to stimulate growth. No mention of the fact that both arsenic and lead are poisons, and no follow-up on what to do if poisoning should occur.

In Queen Victoria's time, hemp was used for menstrual cramps and the growth and development of a stately bosom, according to the LADIES GAZETTE. Commonly known as marijuna, hemp was shredded and put into vats of boiling water, steeped like tea,and rubbed into the skin. Drinking this herb was supposed to be almost as effective as the hot water rub.

One of the most popular bust developers was a cream made of miraculous vitamins and minerals which was sold through catalogs in the 1890's. Its major ingredient was orange juice, since Vitamin C was considered a vital growth supplement.

In more recent times, women by the thousands have answered ads in magazines promising more beautiful bustlines overnight. For only $9.95 , $21.95 or $49.25 they were invited to order a variety of gadets, creams and exercise programs. The problem was, none of them worked.

The only way to increase the bust is through proper diet and exercise. Nothing external can cause growth. Exercise cannot increase the size of the breast itself. Exercise, however, can firm the bust, tone it, increase its size and provide an improved appearance in as little as one month.

This book is designed to help women select the right kind of exercise program for themselves, and carry it through. No magic creams, expensive machines, fancy gadgets or shots are needed. All you need for a more beautiful bustline and a better figure is the determination and willpower to sweat a little as you work at home to develop your bust to its full potential.

Muscles aren't the desired effect, and the exercise in this book will not change a feminine shape into a Mr. Universe body. To begin with, women have a natural layer of extra fat which keeps them from developing hard, masculine muscles. Secondly, the exercises in this book have been used successfully by hundreds of women over a 10 year period and have been refined, adapted and revised based on their experiences until they are a fine art. These exercises build the bust. Only that. They won't turn Twiggy into a sweater girl over-night, but they will work. Most women can expect to see results in a month, with permanent firmness and increased bust size in about 90 days.

INTRODUCTION

For over ten years, I have been involved in the health field serving as a manager, and supervisor of various health spas and clubs. I have also been a director of Dr. S. Cottens Sports Medicine Clinic of Dallas.

During that time I found that while most women seemed to want to build their busts, most did not know how. Their minds were full of questions and problems. They had heard about various exercises and machines, but weren't sure if any of these things would really work.

I have always assured them that while it was not possible to build the breast itself, it was entirely possible to build the bust area (the area around the breast) and to firm and tone the breast and bust area. I then showed them various exercises and machines which would do just that.

Almost without exception, those who followed my program increased both their cup size and bust size dramatically, often as much as several inches in a very short period of time. Because I have run so many different spas and have worked with so many different machines and exercises, I decided to write this book which for the first time, details the **38** ways to increase bust size.

Each one of the exercises is different and will "work" a different part or area of the bust. I assure you that if all are used, the results after three months would be large--perhaps too large. The ideal program incorporates 10 or so of the exercises for three months. Then, after the desired size and firmness is obtained, it can easily be maintained by a few exercises a day.

Women need not worry about becoming too muscular on this program, although excellent muscle tone will be developed by these exercises. What will happen is that the bust and chest area will grow larger and much firmer, and will feel toned and very firm. Women have a natural extra layer of fat which protects their bodies from developing the muscular look and feel which a man would develop on the same program.

The program is easy to follow, requires few "props" or mechanical aids, and can increase overall physical fitness while developing the bust and chest area. Read the directions for each exercise carefully, and the desired results should be achieved within 90 days.

EXERCISE NUMBER 1   REGULAR PUSH UPS

EQUIPMENT NEEDED: NONE

DIRECTIONS:

Place the palms on the floor about shoulder width apart.The back should be kept straight with the knees on the floor. Slowly lower yourself to the ground until your chest touches the floor.

Hold this position for several seconds, then push back up to the original position.

Repeat this exercise 8 to 15 times, increasing the number daily as strength and endurance grows.

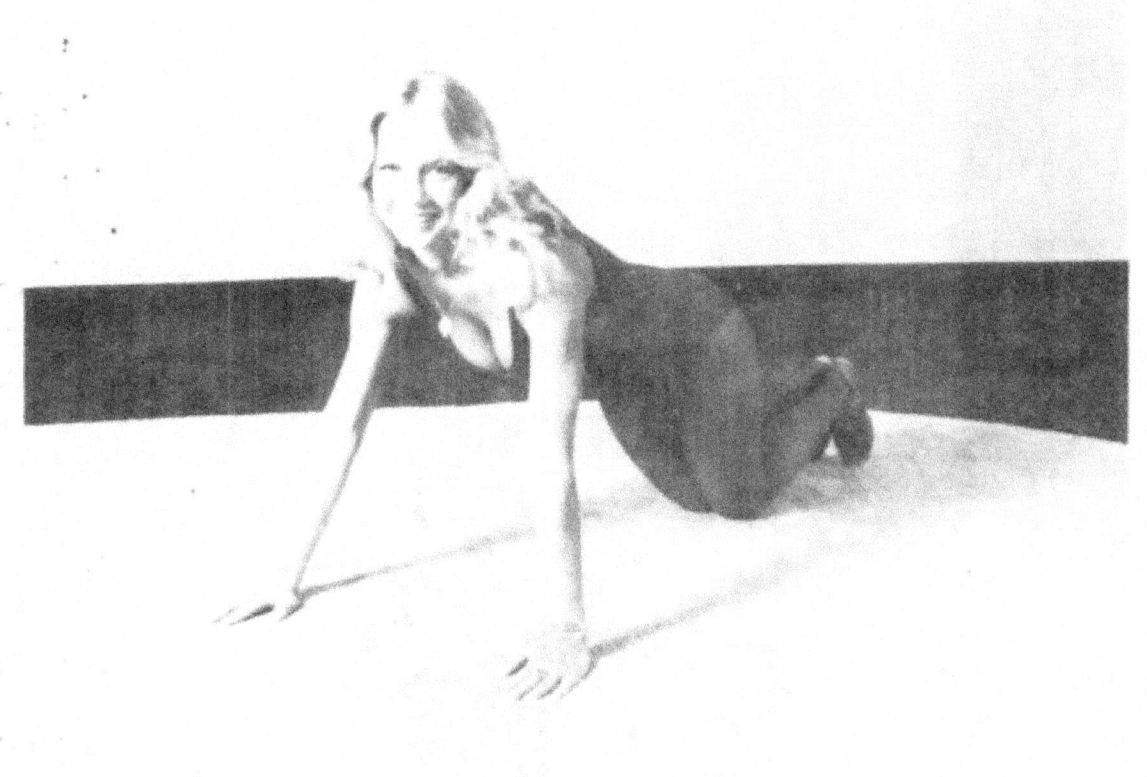

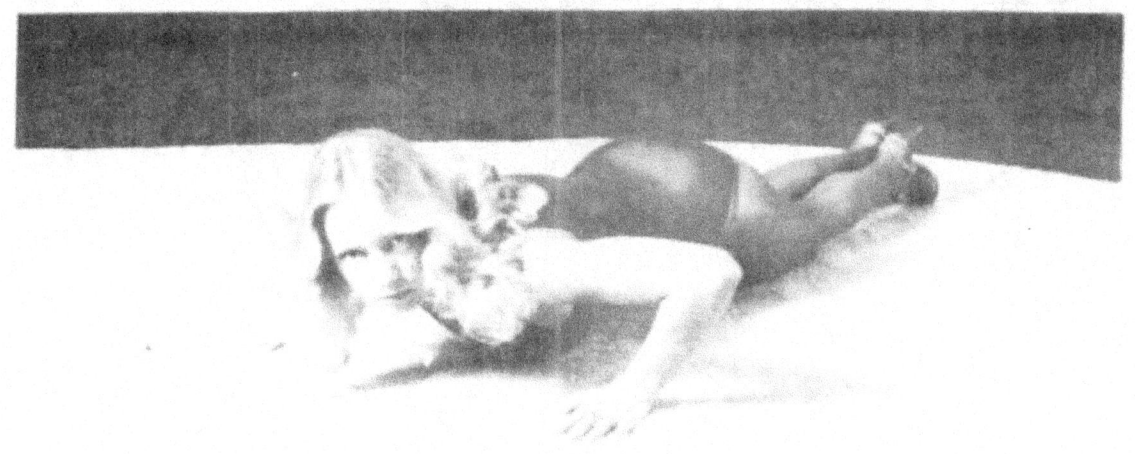

EXERCISE NUMBER 2   WIDE PUSH UPS

EQUIPMENT NEEDED: NONE

DIRECTIONS:
     Place the palms on the ground with the arms extended to about twice shoulder width. Keep the back straight and the knees on the floor. Slowly lower the body down till the chest touches the floor.
     Hold this position at least three seconds, then return to the starting position by pushing slowly back up.
     Repeat 8 to 15 times.
     The wide grip push up exercises the muscles on the sides of the pectoral area and the tops of the breast area.

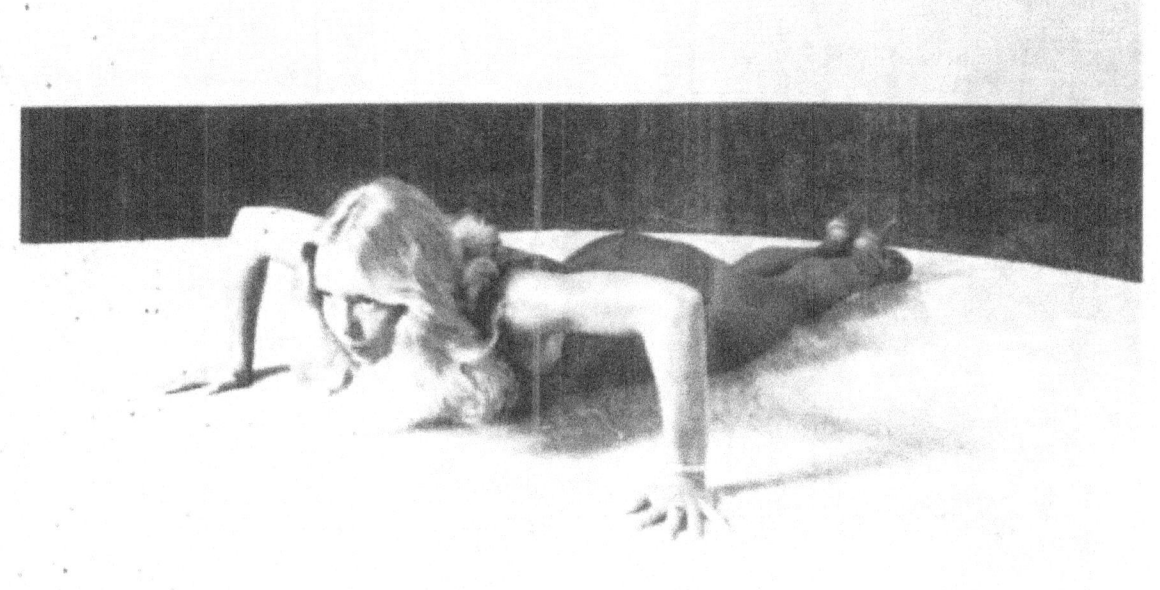

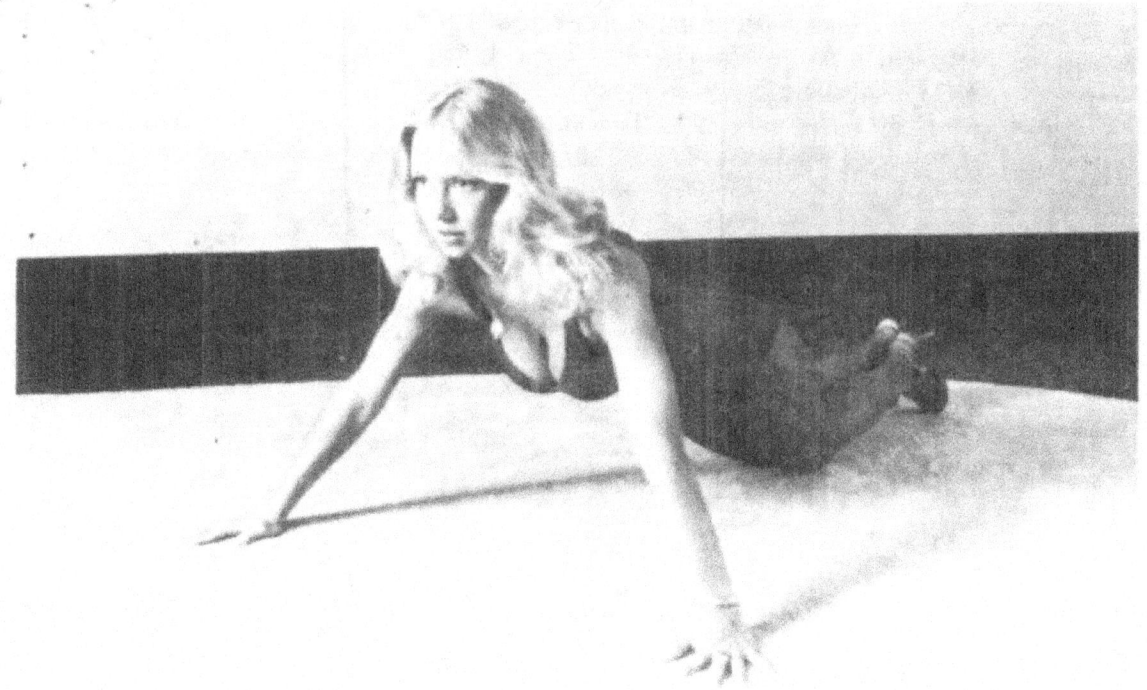

EXERCISE NUMBER *3:*   "V" PUSH UPS

EQUIPMENT NEEDED: NONE

DIRECTIONS:
Place the palms together to form a small triangle directly under the chest. Keep the back straight and the knees on the floor. Slowly lower the body to the ground until the chest touches the hands. Hold this position for three seconds, then push back up to the original position.
Repeat 8 to 15 times.
NOTE: Although these push ups may look somewhat similar. They all work a different area of the chest and when doing them correctly one can easily feel the different chest muscles being exercised.

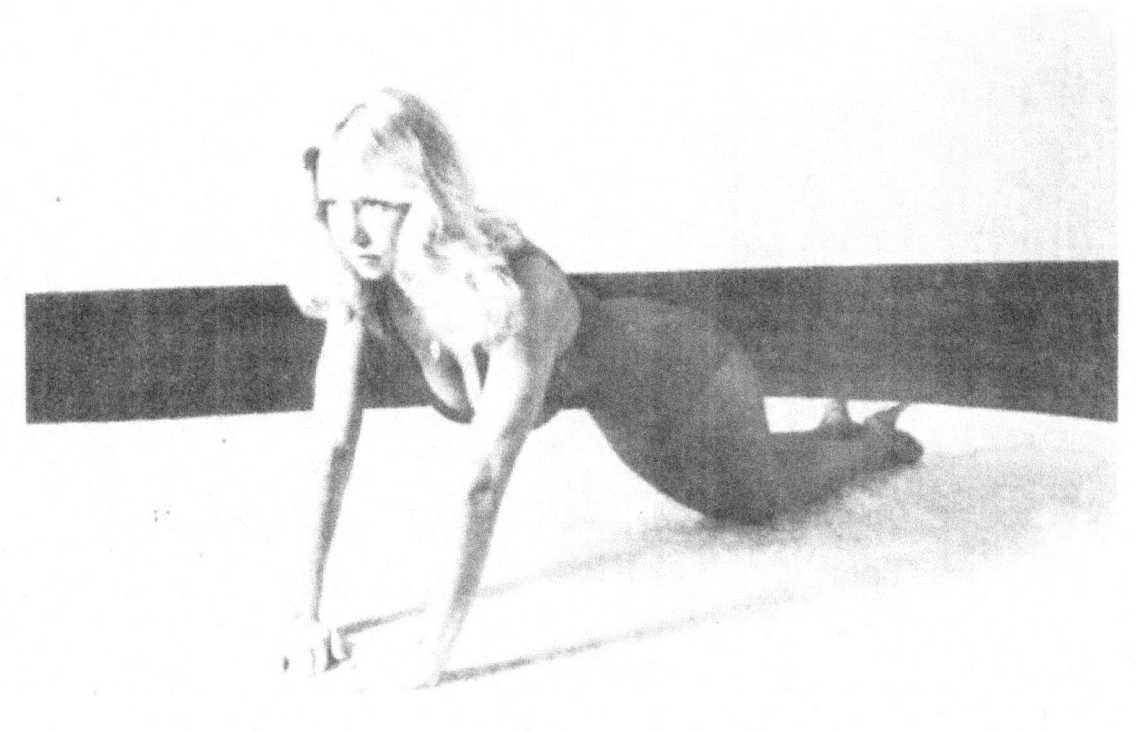

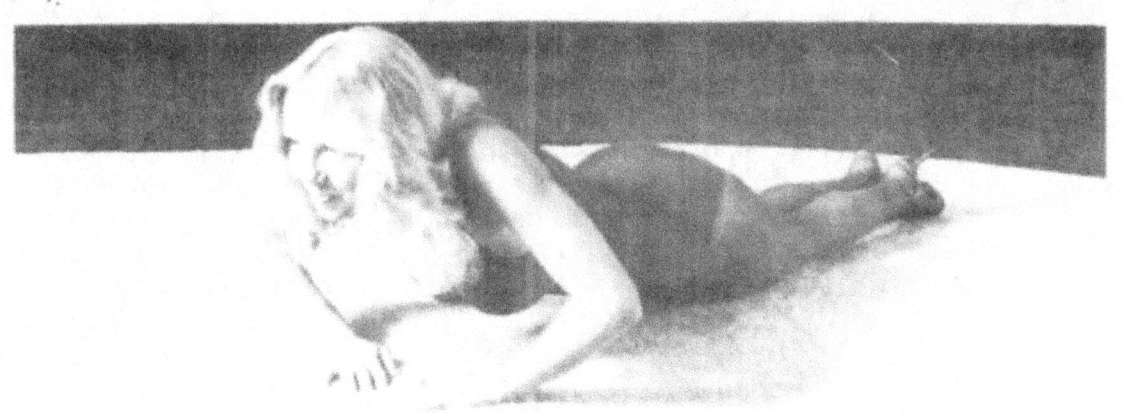

EXERCISE NUMBER 4:   PUSH-UPS BETWEEN CHAIRS

EQUIPMENT NEEDED: Two exercise benches, or two chairs with non skid legs.

DIRECTIONS:
    This variation is more difficult than regular push-ups, but gives better results.   Place two chairs about shoulder width apart, making sure that they are well secured and will not slip Assume the regular push up position, or place the knees on the ground. Using the two chairs, rather than the floor for leverage, slowly lower your body until your chest is at the level of the chairs' seat or slightly lower.
    Hold this position a few seconds, then return to the starting position. Repeat 8 - 15 times.   CAUTION: do not strain on the first few trys...it takes time to build the muscles enough to make this exercise comfortable. As you feel the muscles stretch, continue the exercise only so long as the stretch is only a slight, enjoyable, strain   If it hurts, settle for a push-up which is not so deep.

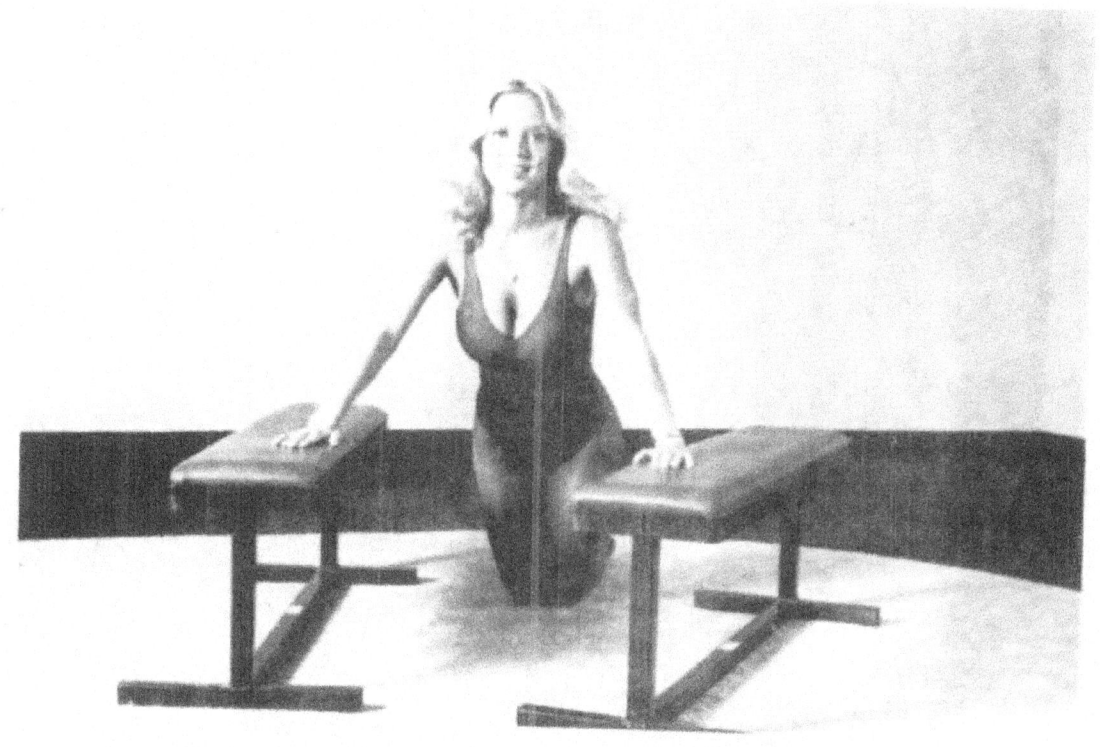

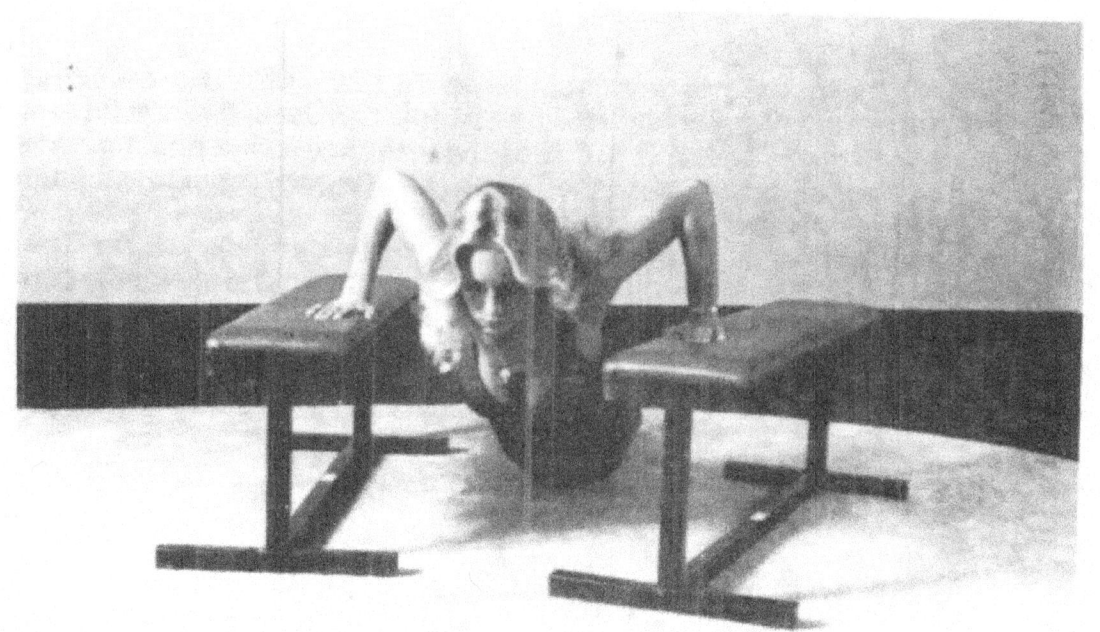

EXERICSE NUMBER 5:　　　**ISOMETRIC PUSHES**

EQUIPMENT NEEDED:　　　**NONE**

DIRECTIONS:

Start with the feet shoulder width apart and the arms directly out in front of the chest. Hold the palms together in front of the body and begin to squeeze the arms together again and again pushing as hard as possible on the palms, as if trying to push the hands completely through each other.

Repeat 8 times, and be sure to concentrate on the chest muscles throughout the exercise. You should be able to feel the bust move as the exercise is being done.

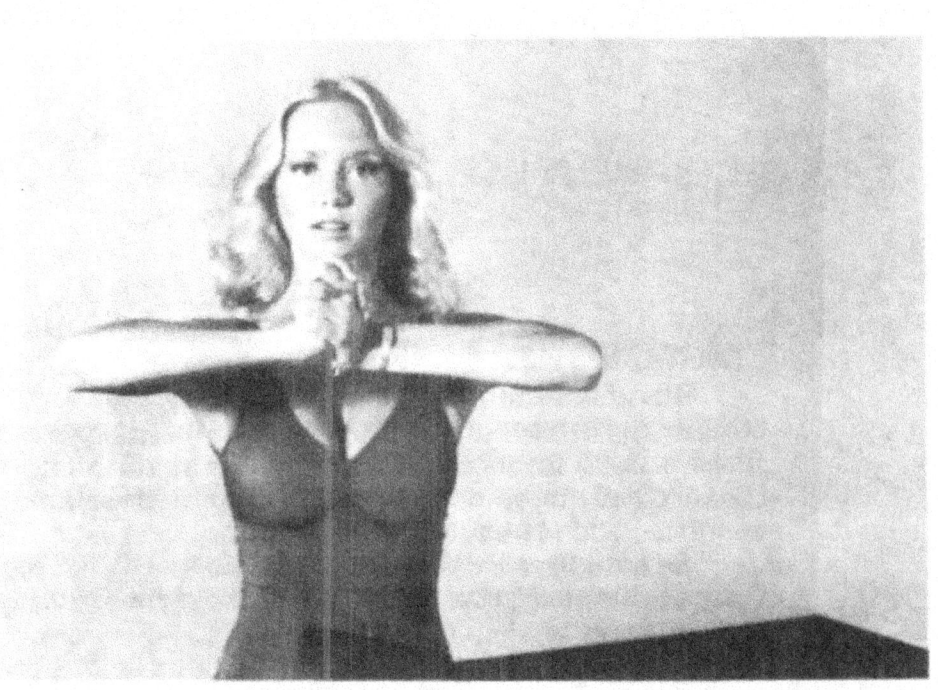

EXERCISE NUMBER 6:   ISOMETRIC PULLS

EQUIPMENT NEEDED: NONE

DIRECTIONS:

Stand with the feet shoulder width apart and hold the arms straight out in front of the chest with the hands grasping each other. Take a deep breath, and pull as hard as possible on each hand, trying to pull the hands apart. Do the pull for 8 seconds, then rest 12 seconds, and repeat three times.

Be sure to pull as hard as possible for the full eight seconds, if you can. It helps if someone counts the eight seconds aloud during the exercise.

This will help to develop the fullness of the bust and is very easy to do.

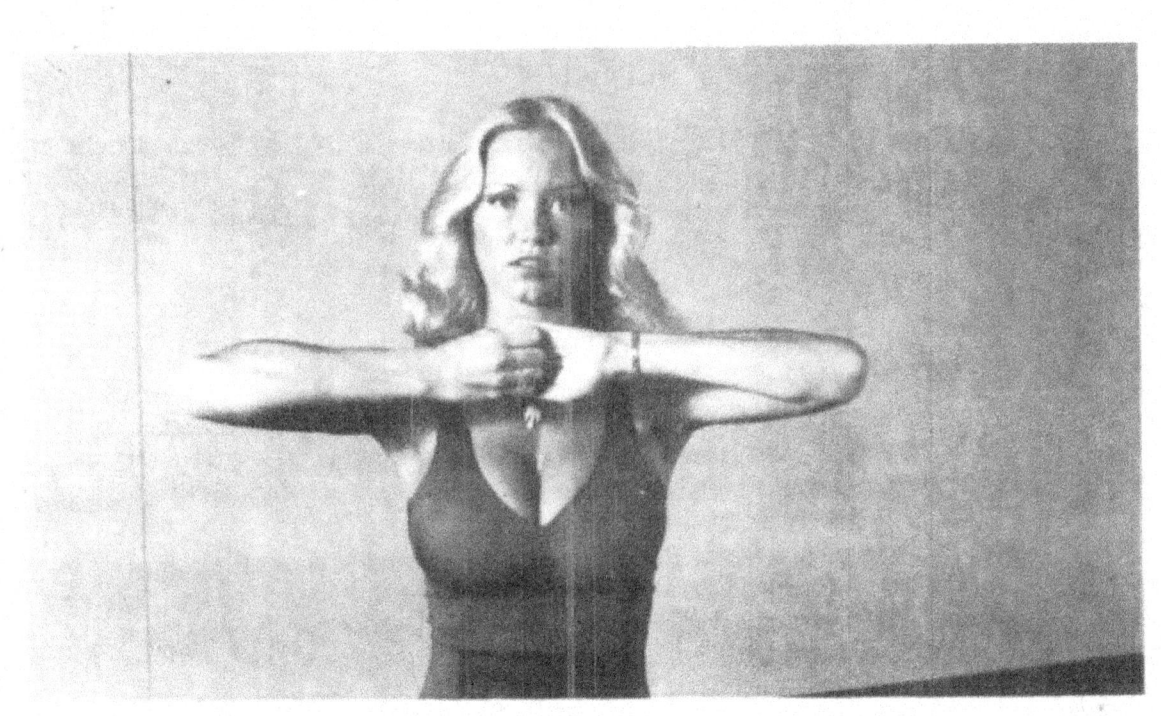

EXERCISE NUMBER 7:   BALL SQUEEZE

EQUIPMENT NEEDED: Small pliable tennis ball or handball

DIRECTIONS:

Stand with the back straight and the arms extended in front of your body, holding a small ball between your palms. Keep the arms slightly bent, and the fingers extended, begin to pump or squeeze the ball between the hands.

You should feel the bust or chest muscles working during the exercise. Repeat 20 - 30 times.

Be sure to concentrate on the muscles in the chest for maximun results.

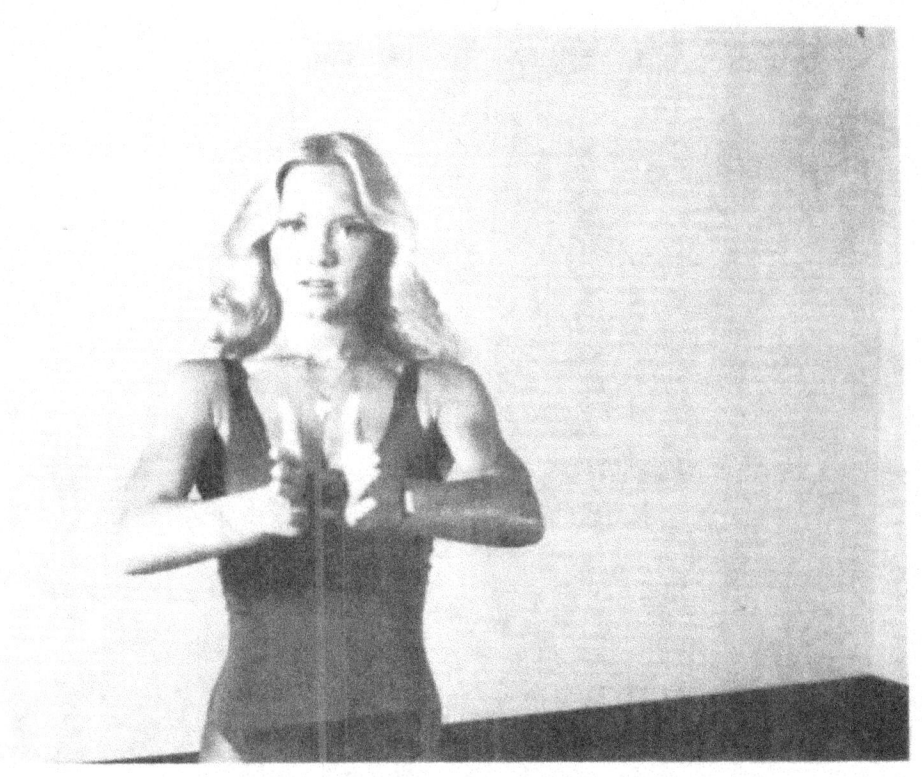

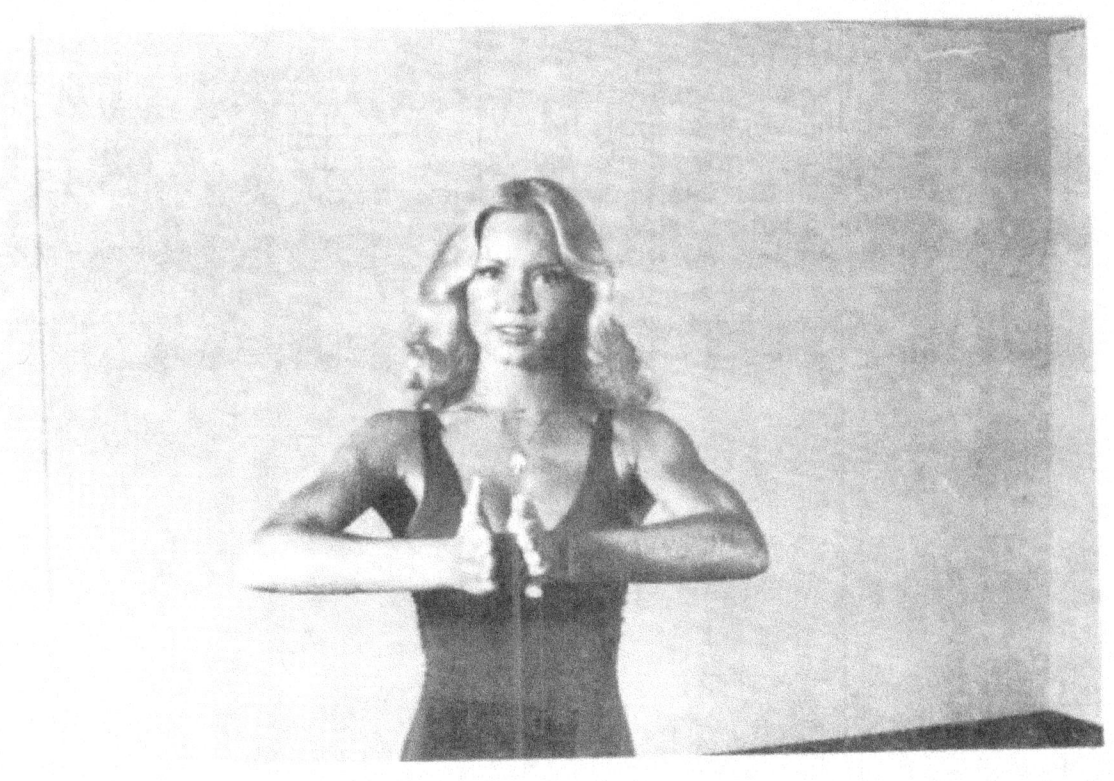

EXERCISE NUMBER 8:   PUSH OFFS FROM THE
                          WALL

EQUIPMENT NEEDED: NONE

DIRECTIONS:
    Lean your body over, stand slightly more than arm's length from the wall, keeping the back straight until the palms rest at shoulder height on the wall. Lower the body slowly towards the wall, until you can move no closer without moving your feet.
    Hold this position a few seconds, then push off the wall to the original position. Results from this exercise increase if you move closer and closer to the wall with each repetition, keeping the elbows level with your shoulders, extended to the left and right.
    Repeat as often as possible, at least 8 - 15 times.

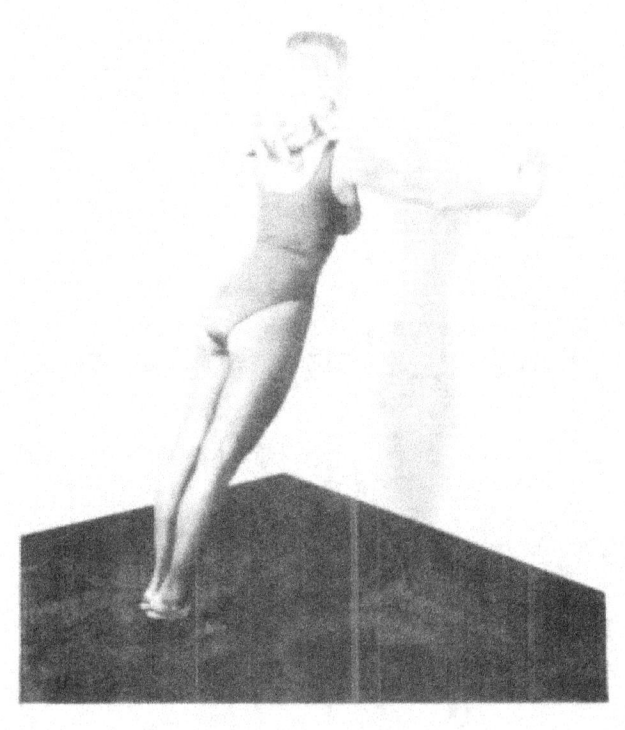

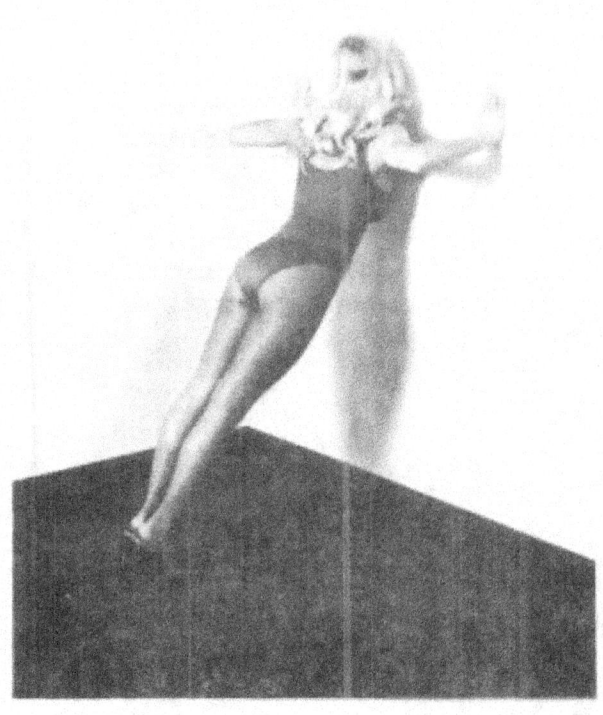

EXERCISE NUMBER 9:   MASSAGE

EQUIPMENT NEEDED: NONE

DIRECTIONS:

Massage is a very useful means of building the bust, because it causes more blood to flow into the chest area. Blood carries protein and enzymes, which can contribute to growth.

It also stretches the tissue and allows for more growth due to the increased size of the tissue.

Hold your breasts in the palm of each hand, and begin to make small but firm, circles on each breast toward the nipples. Always work down from the fullest part of the breast toward the nipples. Alternate hands and breasts. Do this approximately two to five minutes a day.

If a lump or hard cyst is felt in the breast during massage, see a doctor at once.. DO NOT continue the exercise program if a lump is found until your doctor approves your doing so.

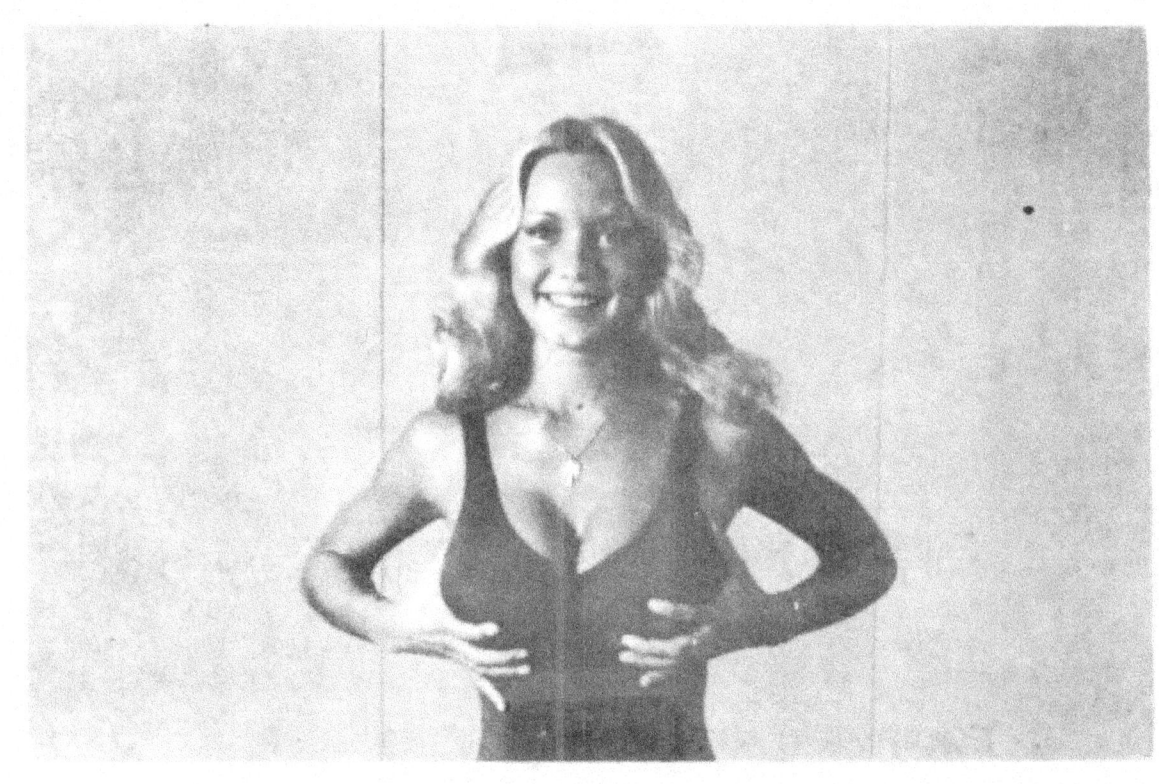

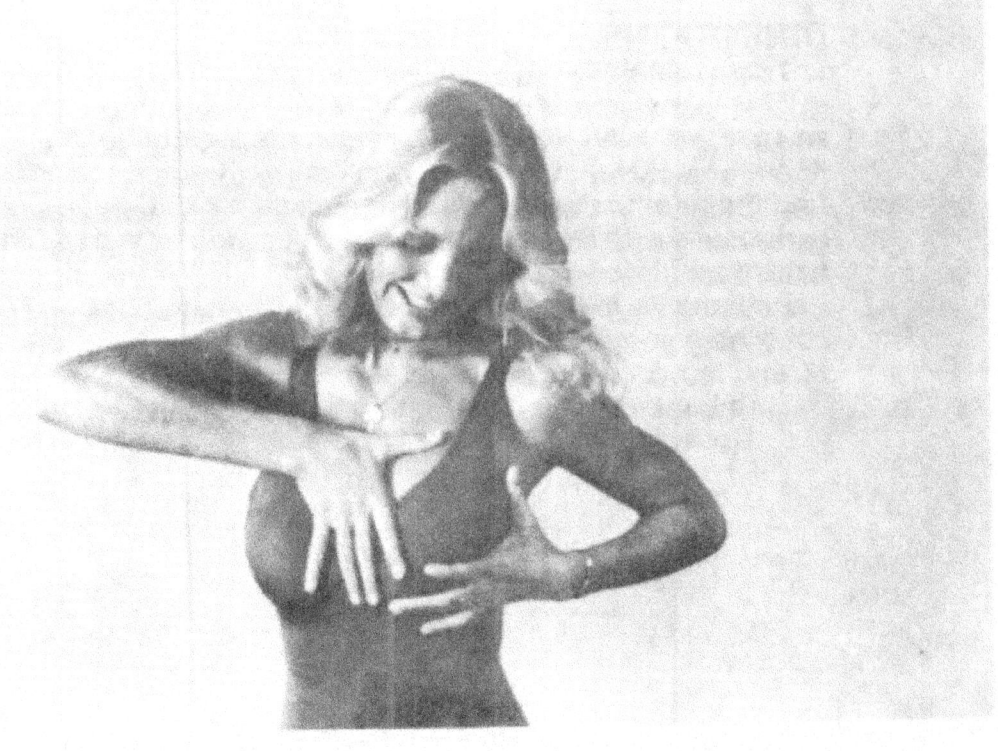

EXERCISE NUMBER 10:   "WE MUST...WE MUST..."

EQUIPMENT NEEDED: NONE

DIRECTIONS:

This exercise is the schoolgirl favorite, commonly done with the rhyme, "we must, we must, we must increase our bust". But it works so well that even women who have left their school days behind find it one of the most effective muscle toners.

Stand with the feet about shoulder width apart and the elbows extended horizontally, to the left and right. Make tight fists with each hand, in front of your chest.

While saying the rhyme, pull vigorously back on the arms, stretching your elbows towards the back as far as they can go-- pulling harder with each repitition.

Repeat 8 times, with each repetition consisting of four "pulls".

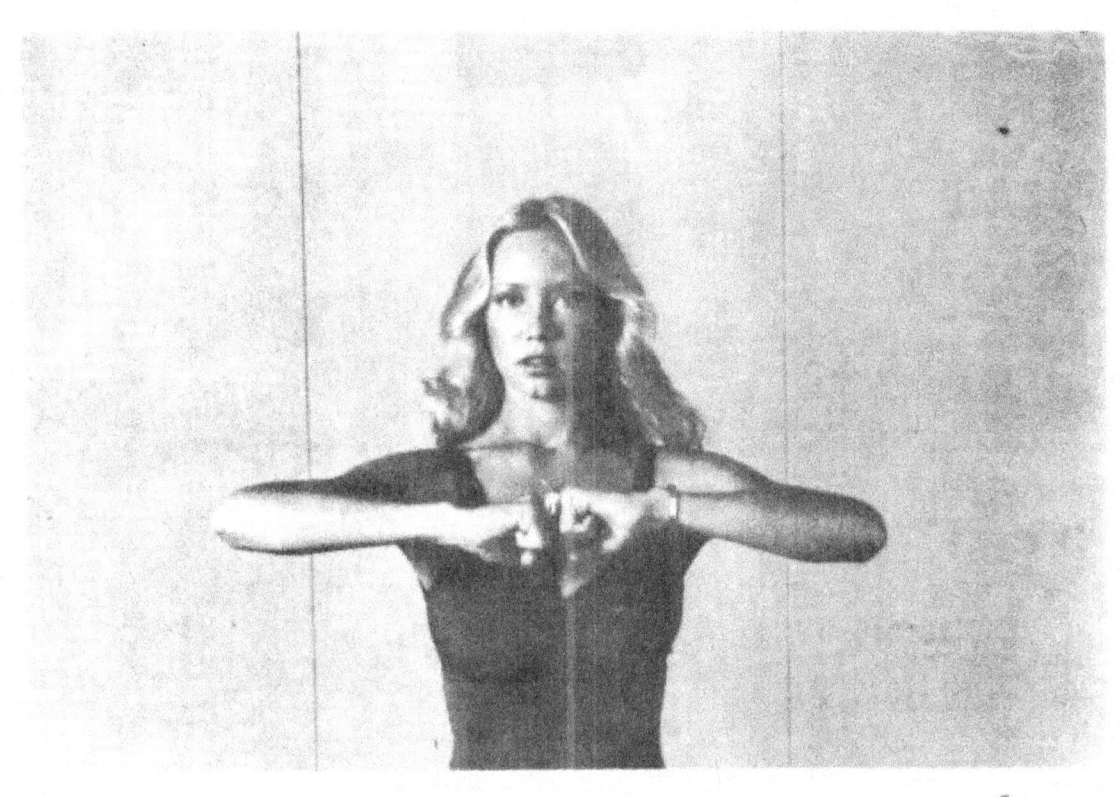

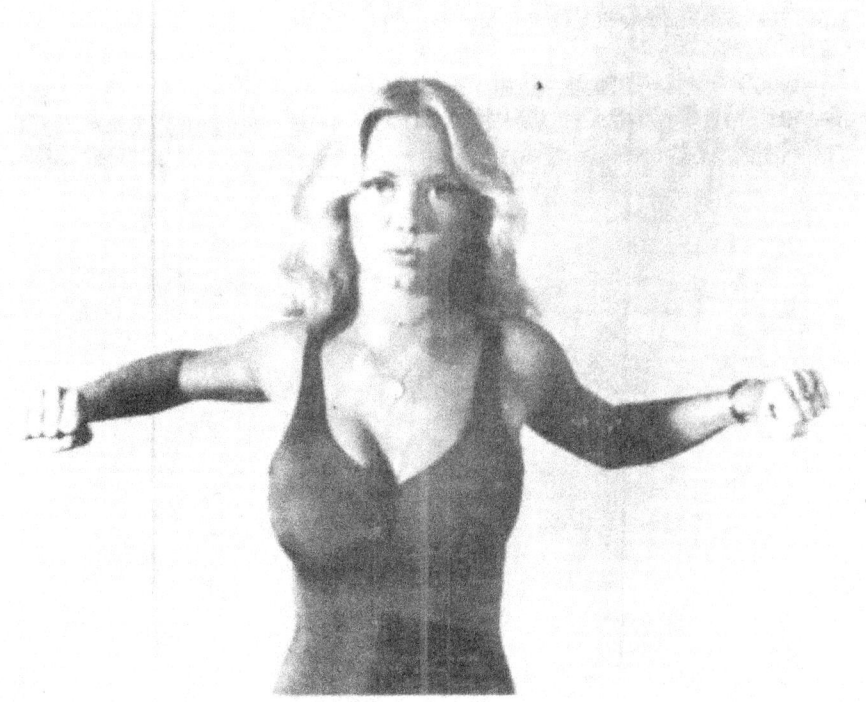

EXERCISE NUMBER 11:   STRETCHES

EQUIPMENT NEEDED: NONE

DIRECTIONS:
    Stand with the feet at shoulder width apart and hold the hands together securely behind the back. Take a deep breath and try to lift the arms up behind the back until they can be lifted no further.
    During the fullest extension possible, the body will be leaning over, and the chest muscles will be stretched to their limit.
    Repeat 8 times, trying to reach higher and higher each time.

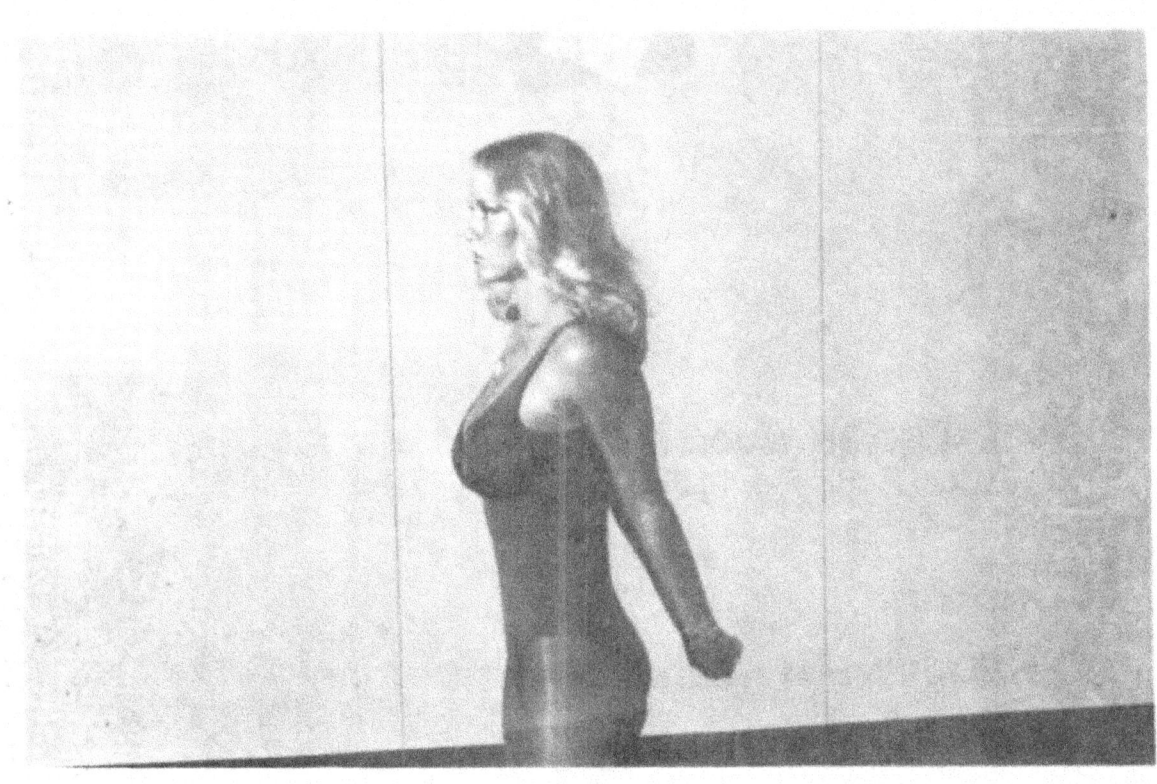

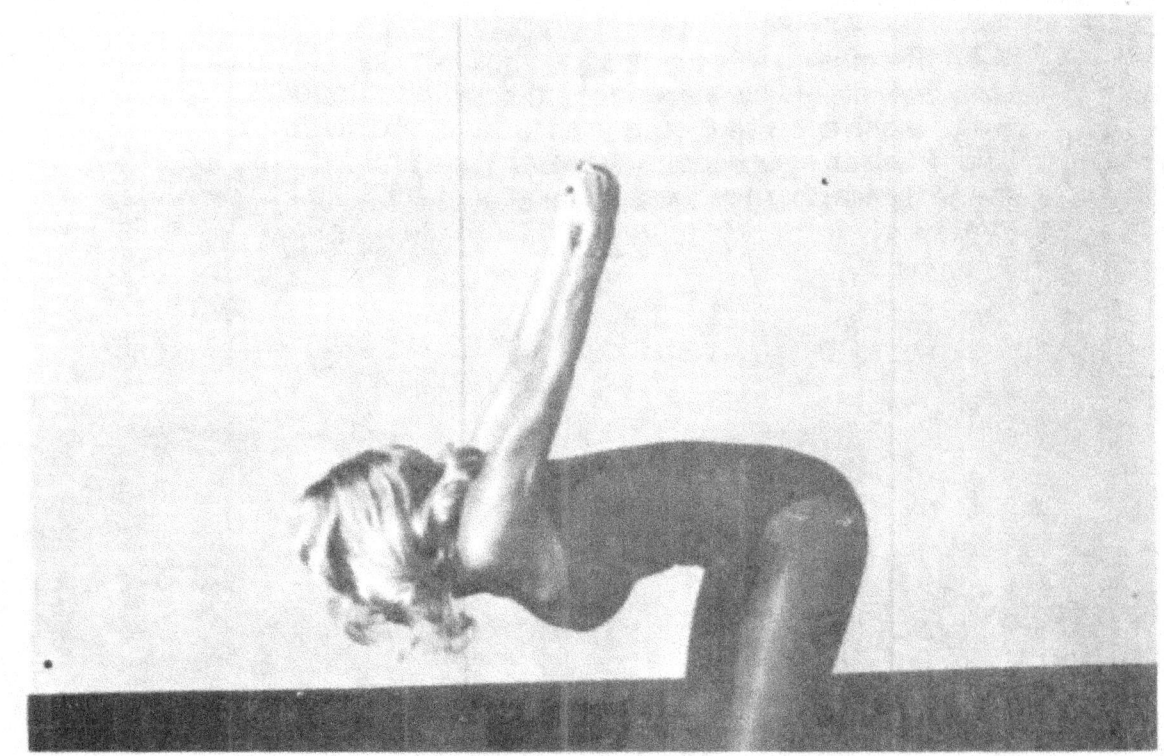

EXERCISE NUMBER 12:   ONE HANDED WALL
                PUSH

EQUIPMENT NEEDED: NONE

DIRECTIONS:
    Sometimes one breast or side of the bust is developed more
than the other....this exercise helps with that common problem.
    Stand a few feet away from the wall and place one palm on the
wall. Use the hand on the side of the LEAST developed breast.
    Push as hard as possible with the palm for eight seconds, rest
for 12 seconds, then repeat the exercise four times.

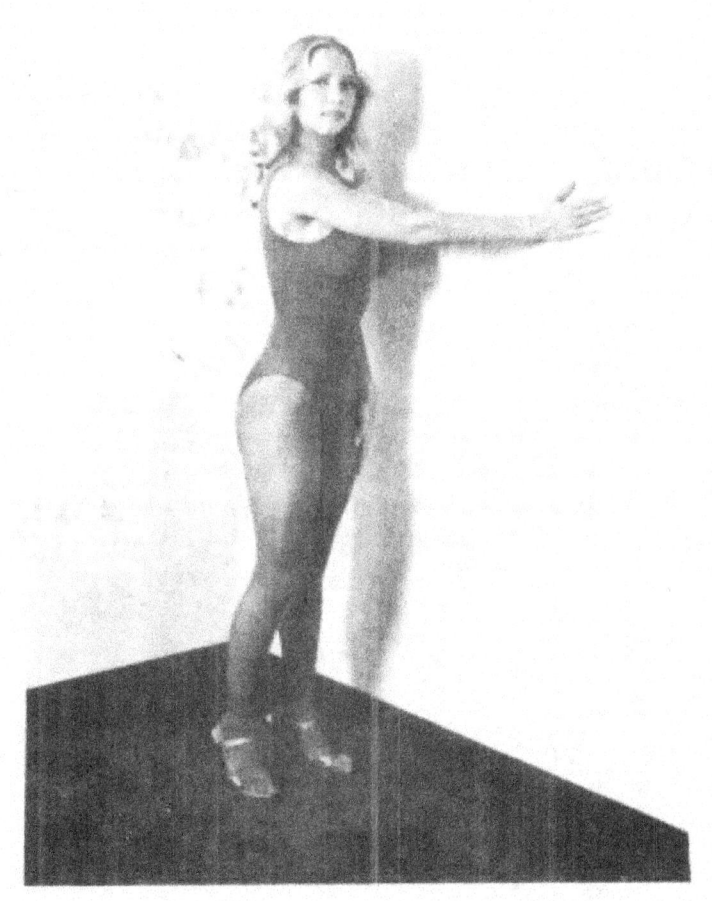

EXERCISE NUMBER 13:   FRONT TOWEL PULLS

EQUIPMENT NEEDED: Terrycloth hand towel or
kitchen towel

DIRECTIONS:
    Stand with the feet apart at the shoulder width holding a towel directly in front of the body at chest height.
    Pull vigorously on the towel for eight seconds, making sure to concentrate on the muscles of the chest. Rest 12 seconds, then repeat three more times.

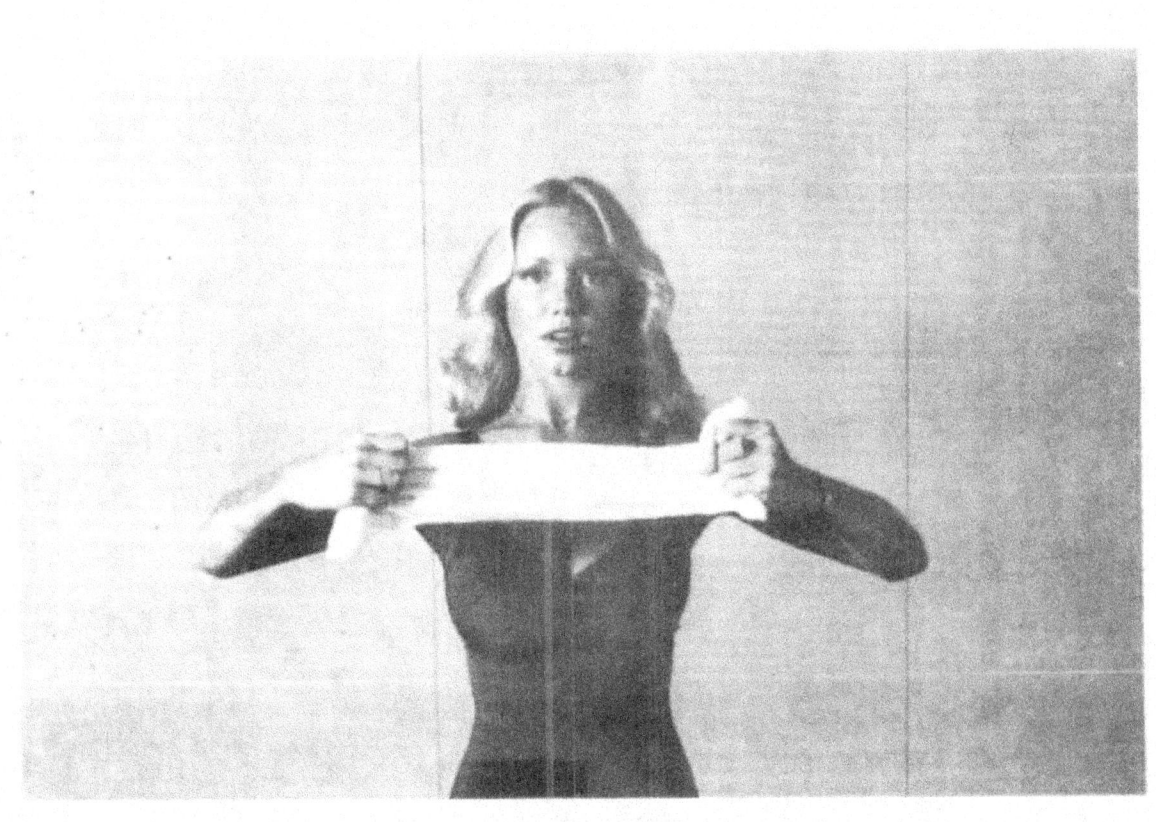

**EXERCISE NUMBER 14:   TOWEL PULLS BEHIND
THE BACK**

EQUIPMENT NEEDED: Terrycloth hand or kitchen
towel

DIRECTIONS:
Stand with the feet shoulder width apart and hold a towel behind the back securely in both hands. Keep the arms as straight as possible and pull vigorously on the towel for eight seconds, making sure to concentrate on the chest muscles while pulling.
Relax for 12 seconds, then repeat three more times.

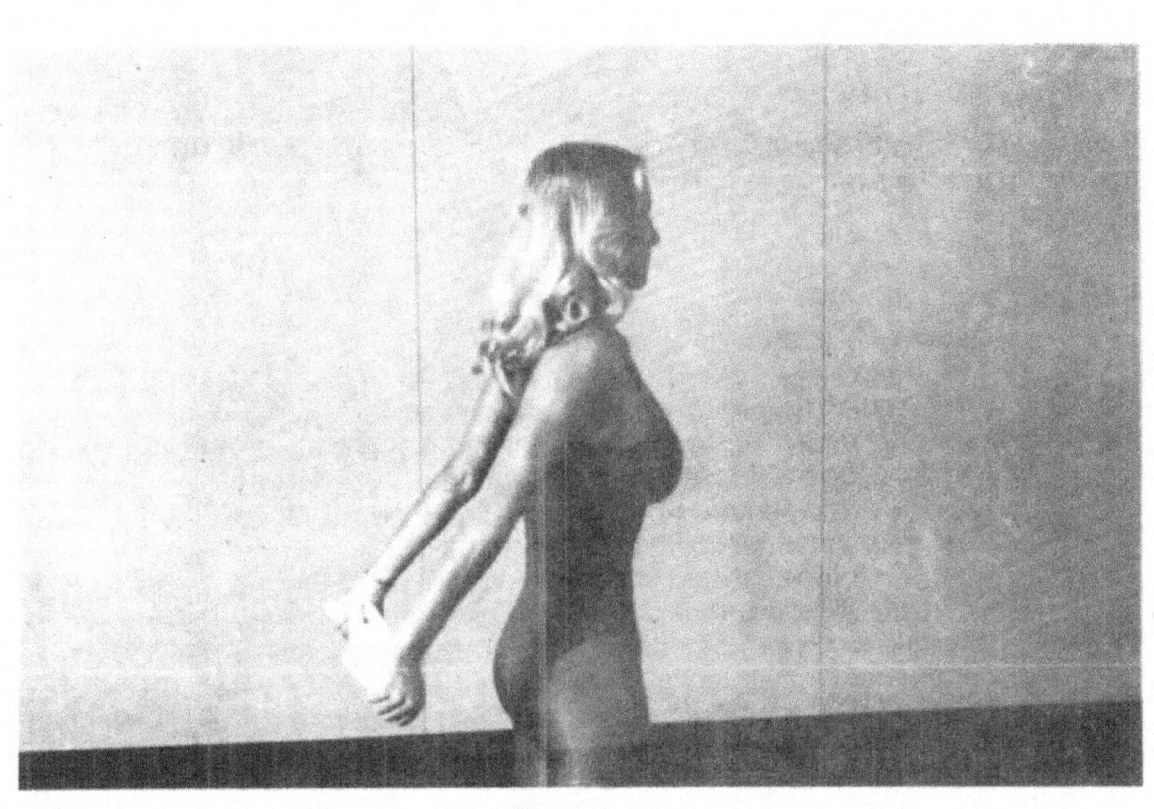

EXERCISE NUMBER 15: COMMERCIAL SPRING EXERCISES

EQUIPMENT NEEDED: Commercial spring-type chest exerciser

DIRECTIONS:

Literally dozens of commercial spring-type chest exercisers are available in sporting goods stores and through mail-order ads in magazines. The two most common are the stretch spring, which looks like two springs connected by two handles, and the "Y" shaped spring, which has hand grips at the bottom and a small, strong spring, at the top

The illustrations show both of the most common devices. No matter what the brand name, all of these devices operate on the same principle: Developing the bust or chest area by providing a set amount of tension. The effect is similiar to that of exercise number 7, the ball squeeze, but is maximized by the strength of the spring.

But pushing against the resistance of the spring provides faster and greater results than either isometric pushes or ball squeezes. When purchasing the springs at a sporting goods store, the clerk should be able to recommend a spring which is not too strong for your build and size.

The most effective way to use the springs is to stand with the feet at about shoulder width and hold the spring between your open palms at chest height. Keeping the palms open, push the springs together as many times as possible. Rest a few minutes between exercises, repeating the sequence of as many quick pushes as possible at least three times.

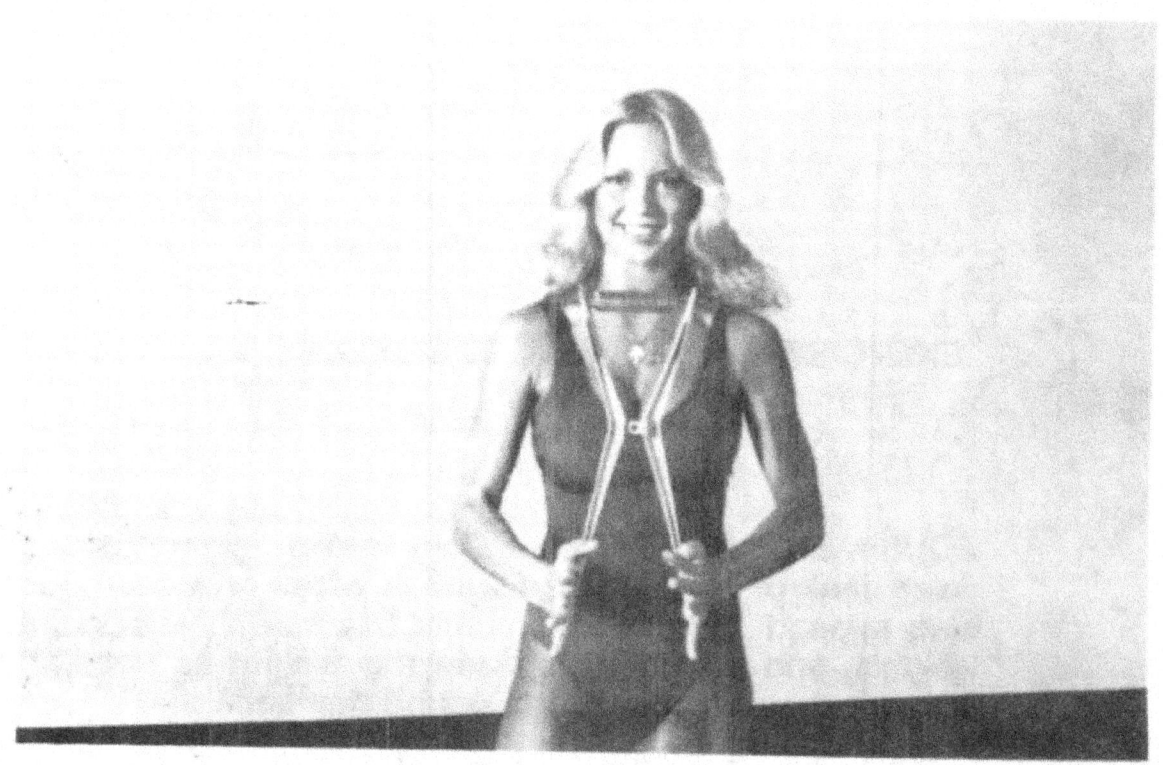

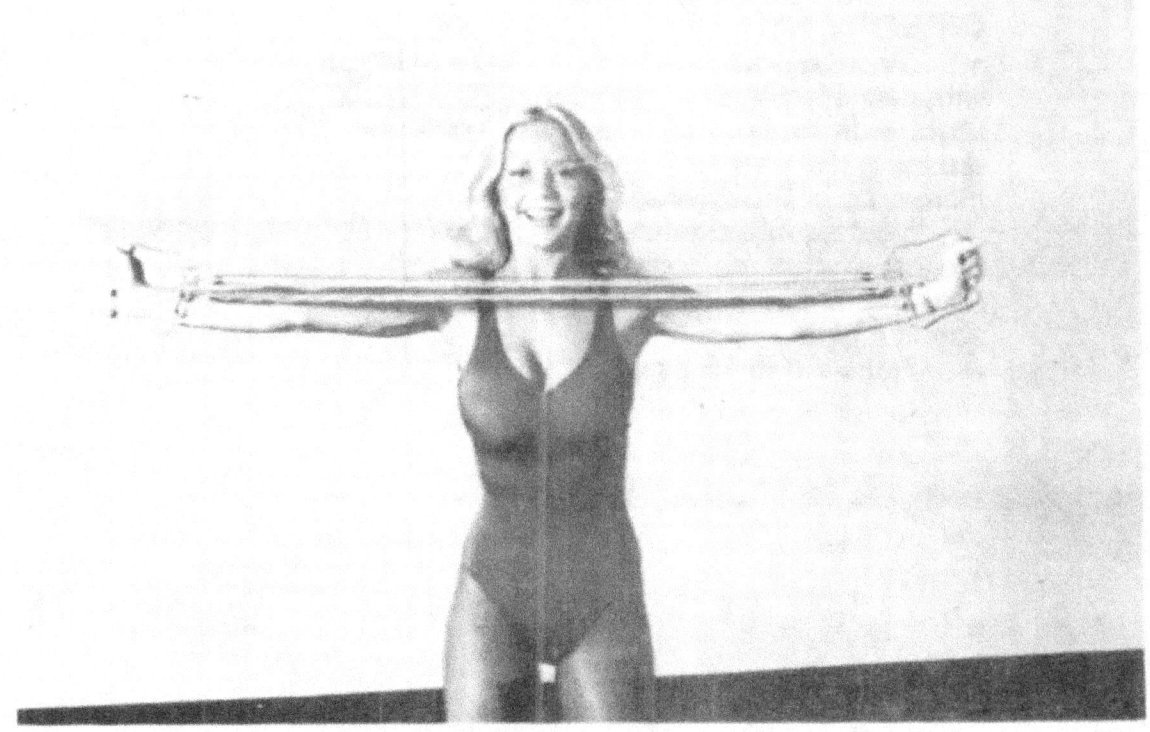

EXERCISE NUMBER 16:   DUMBELLS ON AN INCLINE

EQUIPMENT NEEDED: Commercial incline board, lawn chair or other slanted surface which provides good body support. Two small dumbells(begin with three pound weights, and gradually increase the weight as strength increases), up to about eight pound dumbells.

DIRECTIONS:
Sit on the incline boards holding a pair of dumbells in each hand, with palms facing away from the body. Slowly lower the weights in a slight arch to each side until the arms can go no further without dropping the weights. As strength grows, the stretch widens, thus increasing is effectivenss.
Hold the fully extended stretch for a few seconds, then squeezing the chest muscles together, lift the weights back to the starting position. The exercise may be done with both arms together, or one arm at a time.
Repeat 8 to 15 times.

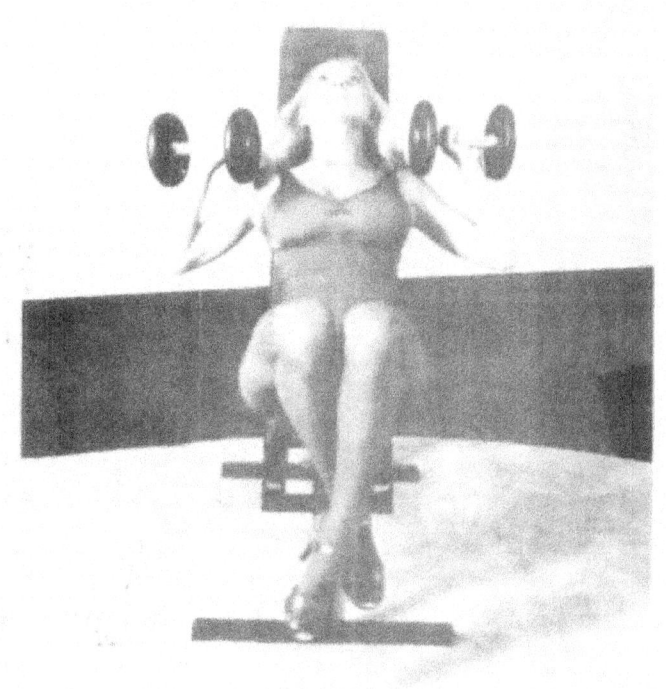

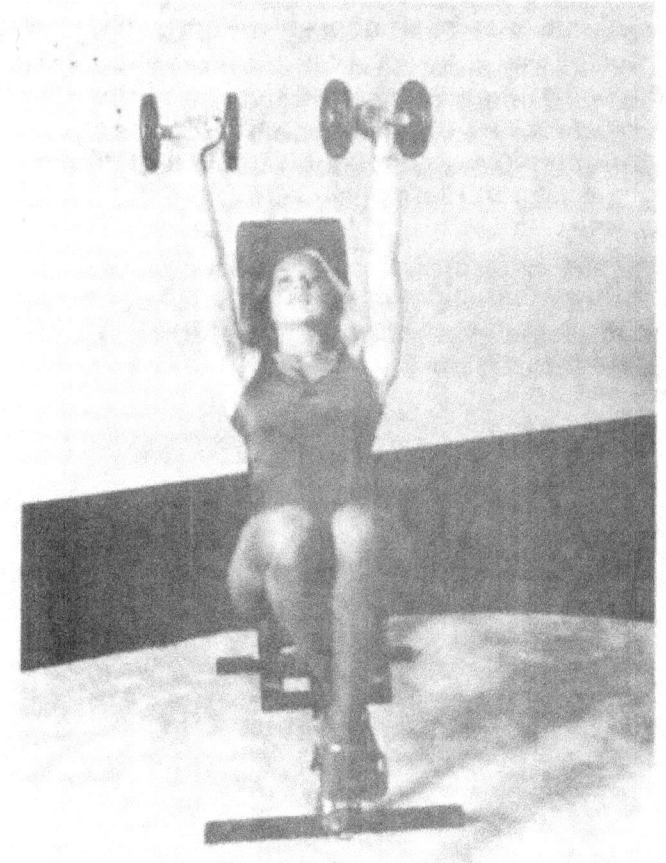

EXERCISE NUMBER 17:   THE FLY

EQUIPMENT NEEDED: Two Dumbells

DIRECTIONS:

This exercise is a basic chest development exercise, and one of a family known as the "flies". Using a flat bench or the floor for this exercise works the muscles on the inside of the chest.

Lie flat on a bench or the floor and hold a pair of dumbells at arm's length, straight above your shoulders. Your palms should face each other as the weights are slowly lowered, in a slight arch, to the sides of your hips, keeping the arms fully extended. DO NOT let the weights touch the floor.

Hold this full stretch for three seconds, then push the weight back to the original starting position. Concentrate on squeezing the chest muscles together during the exercise.

Repeat 8 to 15 times..

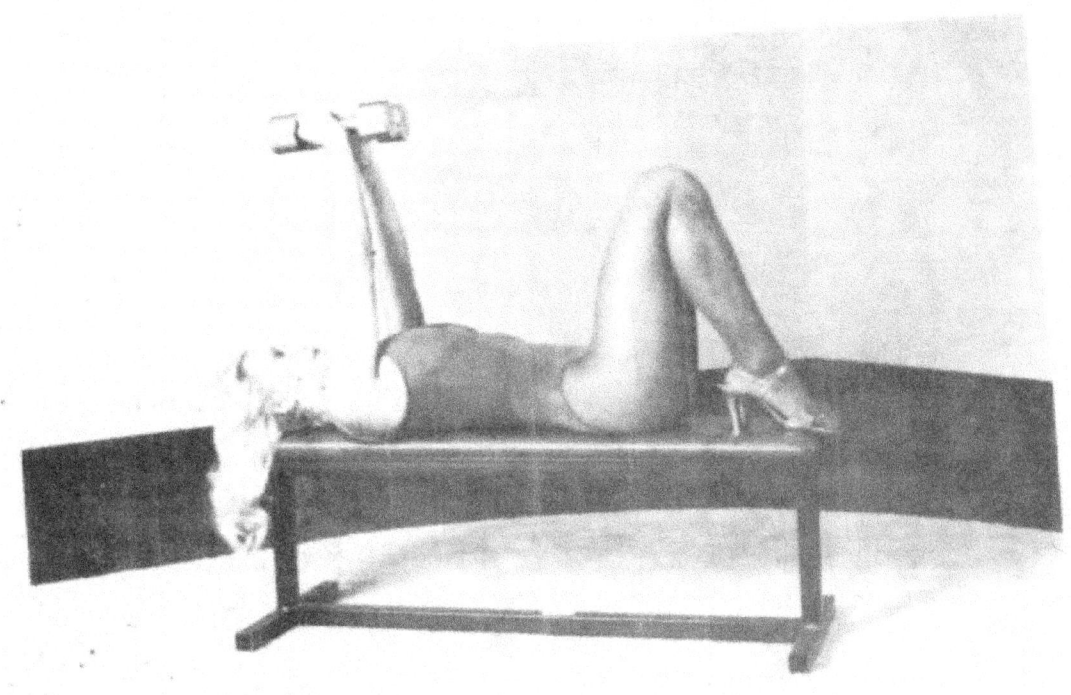

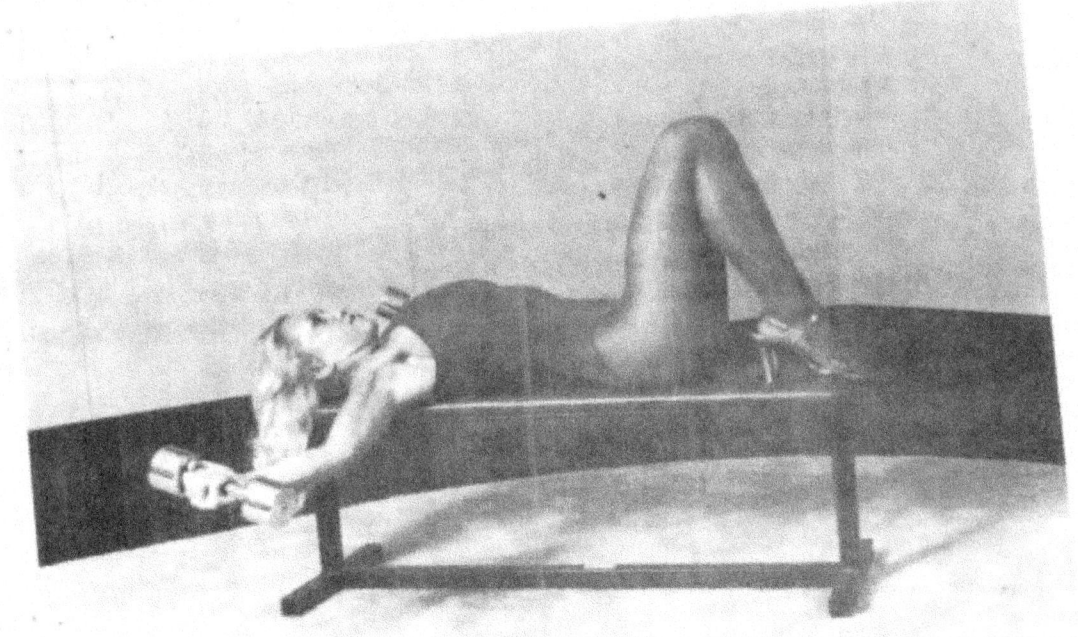

EXERCISE NUMBER 18:   CROSS FLYS

EQUIPMENT NEEDED: Incline board, bench or lawn chair, two dumbells

DIRECTIONS:

Lie flat on a bench and hold a pair of dumbells , arms extended, in the hands directly over the chest. Slowly bring the weights down towards the floor as in the previous two exercises. Keep the arms at a slight arch.

Hold this extension a few seconds, then squeeze the chest muscles together and push the weights back up and across the front of the body into an"X" directly over the chest. This really squeezes the chest muscles together and adds to the development of a fuller chest.

Do not jerk the weights into the "X" , and do not attempt to do this (or any other) exercise using too quick a movement. Slow methodical movements are safer and provide greater results.

Repeat the exercise eight times.

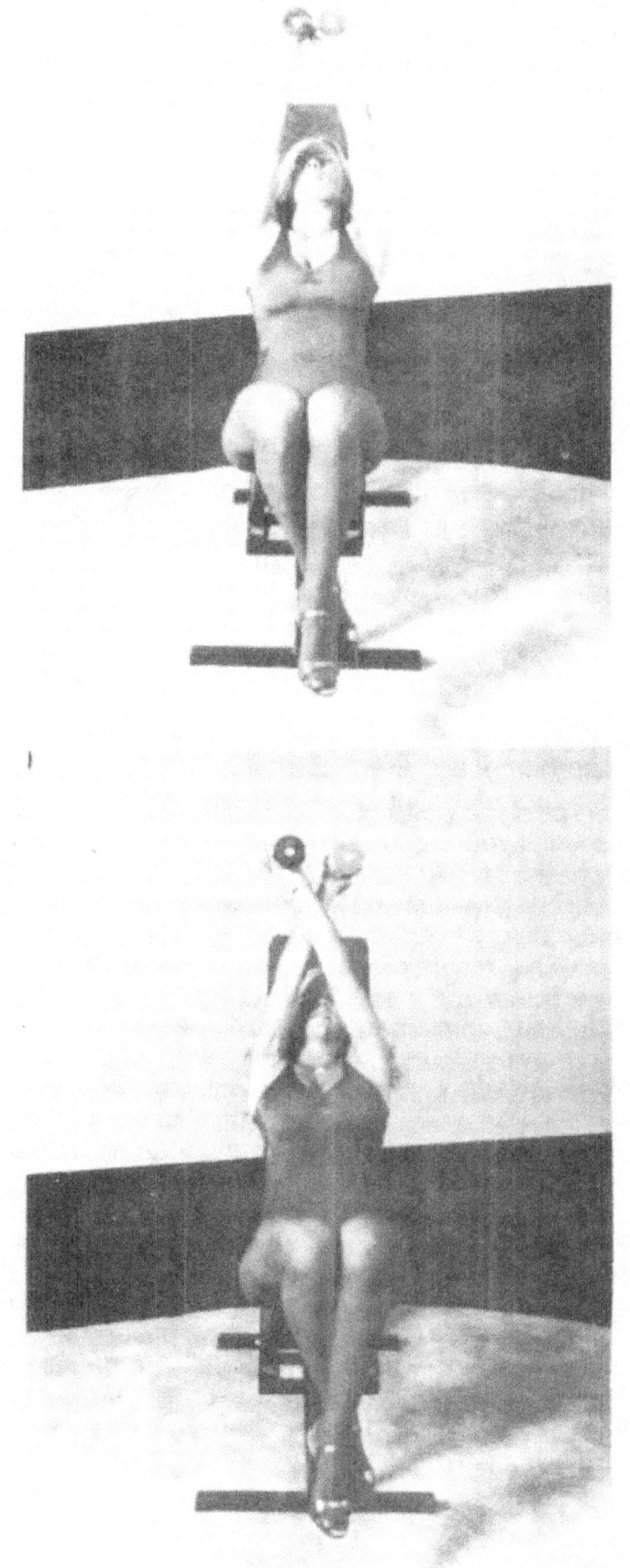

EXERCISE NUMBER 19:   THE BENCH PRESS

EQUIPMENT NEEDED: Barbell (see weight instructions below), bench press bench, or two chairs with non-skid legs. A partner, or spotter.

DIRECTIONS:

Never attempt bench presses or other exercises using barbells without a spotter or assistant. Lie flat on the bench or floor, and have the spotter hand you weights to determine the right weight to exercise with.

The spotter should hand you the weight and help you balance it for a moment before taking his hands away. Should the weight be too heavy, he or she can quickly relieve you of the weight.

To exercise the chest area, use a flat bench or a commerical bench press board and a barbell with a light to medium weight. Lie on your back on the bench and either lift the weight off the bar (or backs of two chairs which support the weight until you are ready for it) or have someone hand it to you. Hold the weight with the arms fully extended and slowly lower the weight down until it touches the chest.

Hold this position three seconds, then push the weight away from the chest and back up to the original position. Do Not lift any part of the body off the bench during the exercise, and keep the weight directly over the chest. Do the bench press eight times.

NOTE: Many health spas and clubs have "bench press machines" which exercise the chest area in the same way as conventional bench press exercises but are safer and easier for the beginner. If you belong to a spa or club, check with their manager for details of using such a machine to develop your bust.

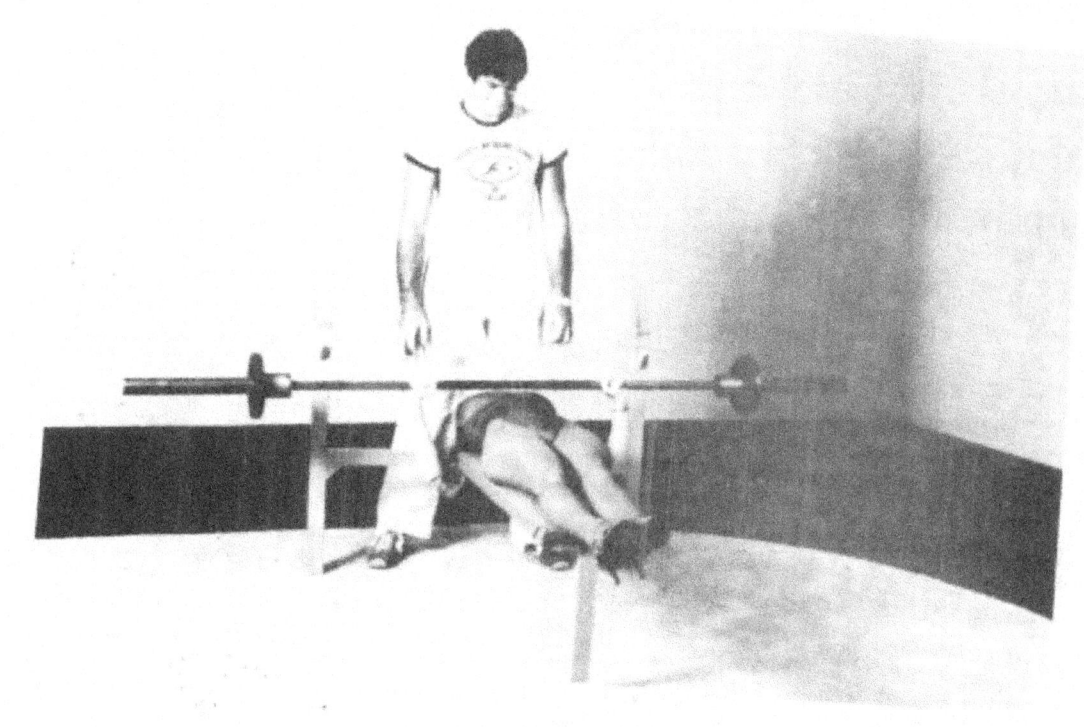

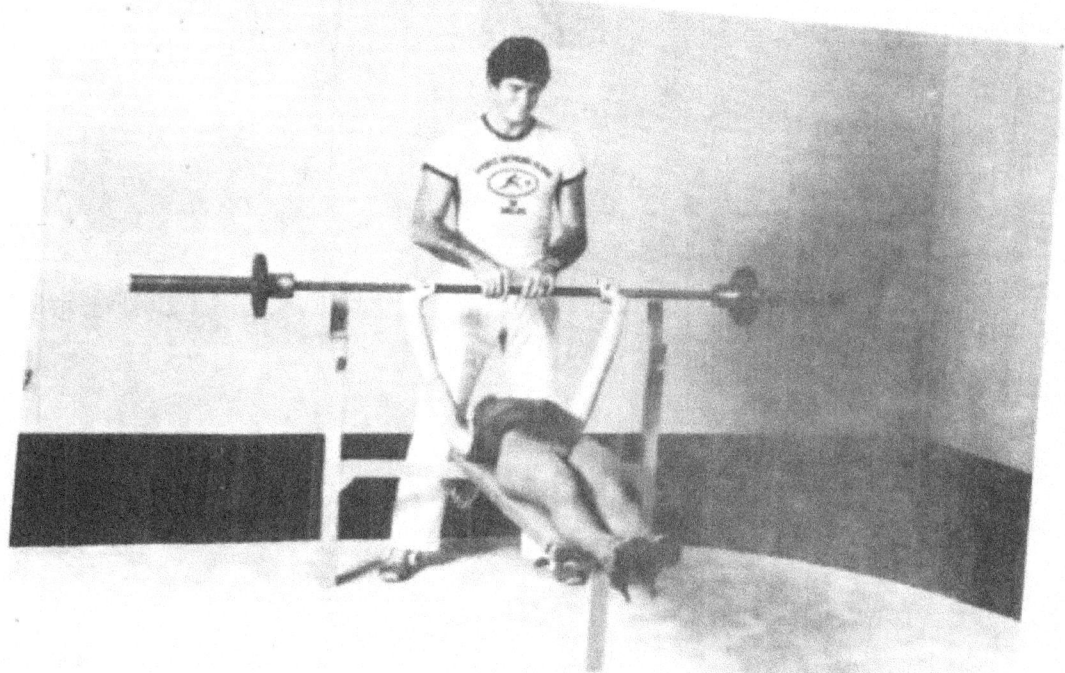

PROTEIN AND DIET CONTROL FOR BUST DEVELOPMENT

Protein is the major source of building material for the body and as such is necessary for all growth to take place. Protein is essential in the formation of hourmones which control such bodily functions as growth and rate of metabolism. It also helps to regulate the body's water balance. It is important in the formation of milk during preganancy, and forms enzymes which are vital for basic life functions. It is responsible for over 80% of muscle mass.

Protein is composed of 22 amino acids, all produced in the body, except for 8 essential ones. Therefore, when considering the purchase of protein supplements, be sure to check the label to see that all of the amino acids are present in the supplement. The necessary amino acids which cannot be synthesized by the human body are:

Isoleucine
Leucine
Lysine
Methionine
Phenylalanie
Treionine
Trypotophan
Valine

Controlling the diet during this exercise program by adding foods which are high in protein such as lean meats, cheese, eggs,and fish, provides the body with the additional protein requirements caused by this exercise program.

The national research council recommends that 0.42 grams of protein be consumed per day for each pound of body weight. A 100 pound woman, in order to assure herself of the necesary protein and amino acids, would have to eat 42 grams of protein per dav. The federal government estimates that the average consumption only 14 grams per day.

Taking protein supplements or following a dietary regime which does not provide all the necessary amino acids is not helpful to a complete growth and exercise program, because the human body is only able to utilize the amino acids in the amount of the acid in the least amount. This means that is the diet or supplement provides 6 grams of all the proteins acids except one, but only supplies 2 grams of it, then the body is only able to utlize 2 grams of any of the other amino acids. All 22 of the acids need to be utliized in equal amounts, so it is important to plan diets or supplement programs carefully.

Most meats and dairy products contain all the necessary amino acids, but most fruits and vegetables do not. A protein supplement plus a balanced diet aids muscle growth, especially in the muscles which are being exercised very hard in this bust development program. Many women have found that taking two or three spoonfuls of protein powder per day helps keep the bust firm and toned and aids in faster development. Naturally any such food supplement program should be approved by your doctor.

EXERCISE NUMBER 21:   DECLINES

EQUIPMENT NEEDED: Dumbells, sit-up board, decline board or upside down lawn chair.

DIRECTIONS:
Using a sit-up board or slanted bench or lawn chair, lie flat on your back with the feet higher than the head. Have someone hold your feet or anchor them on the bar of the sit-up board.

Hold a pair of dumbells directly above the body near the chest with the palms facing outwards. Slowly lower the weights to each side of the body until they can go no further.

Hold the full stretch a few seconds, then return the weights to the original position. Repeat eight times.

This is an exercise which should be done with a comforatble weights rather than the limit of your tolerance. Two-five pound weights are normally used by women in this exercise even if they use greater weights for other exercises.

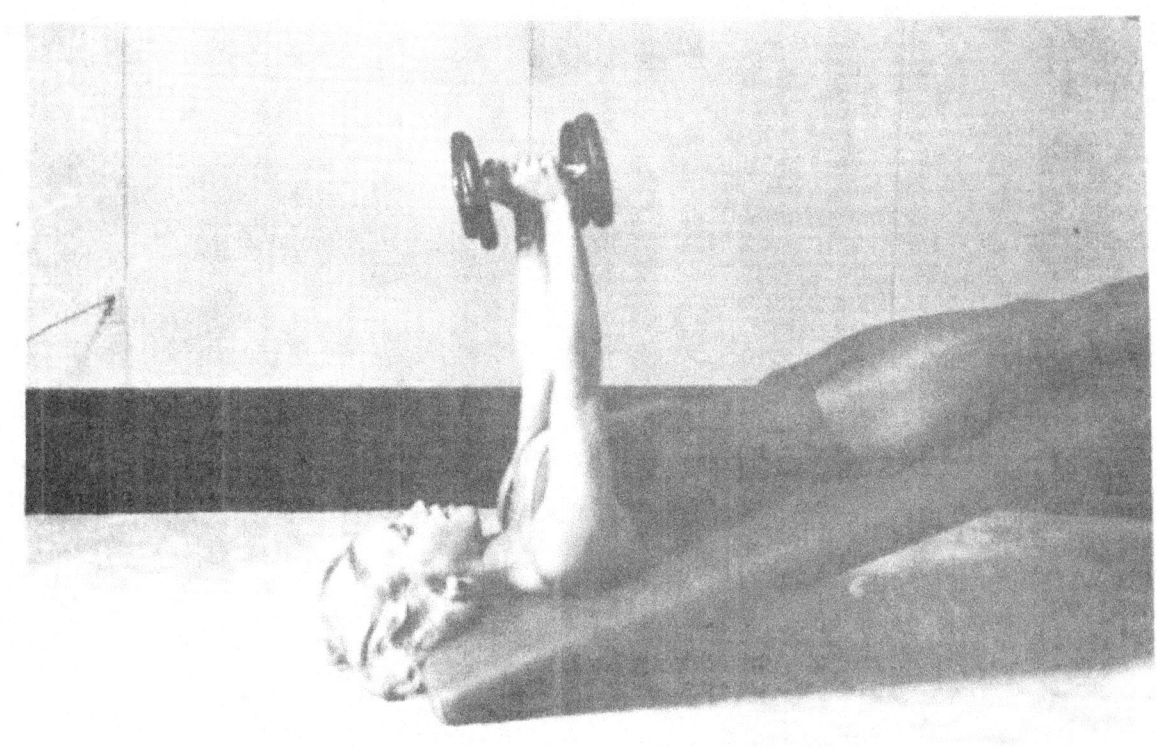

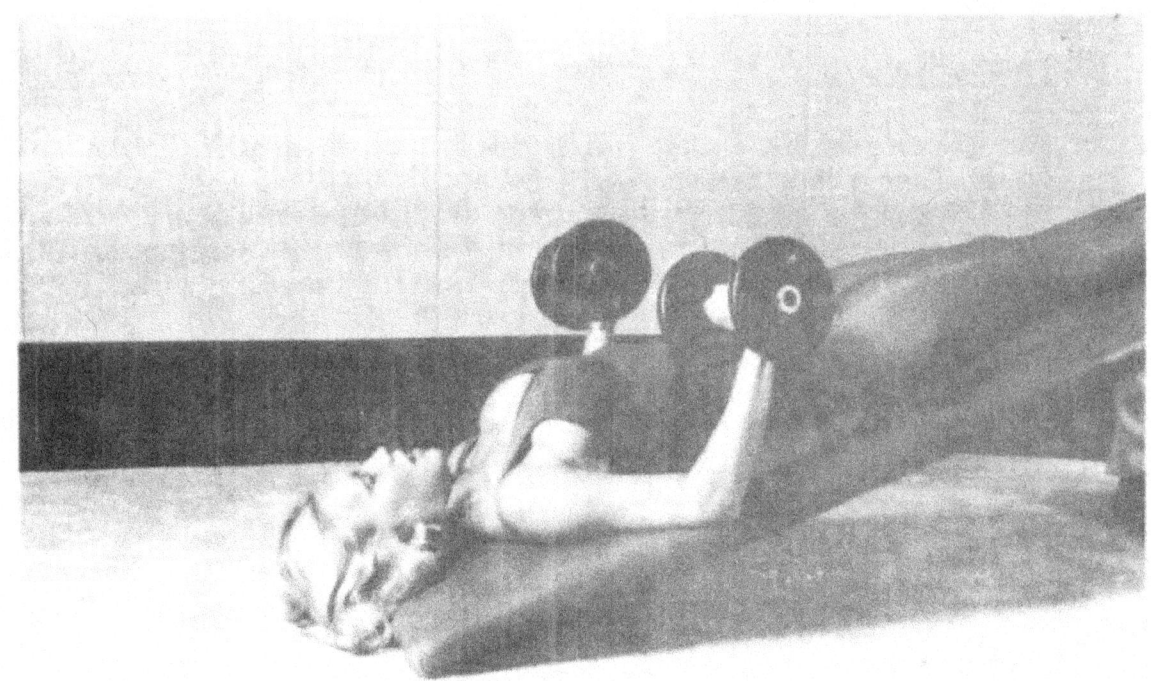

EXERCISE NUMBER 22:   DUMBELL PRESS ON A
                FLAT BENCH

EQUIPMENT   NEEDED: Dumbells, flat bench,
coffee table or two stools

DIRECTIONS:

   Lie on a flat bench with two dumbells at arm's length over the
chest. Take a deep breath, hold it,and slowly lower the weights to
the sides of the body until they are on each side of the chest.
   Hold this position three seconds, then return the weights to
the original position before exhaling. Repeat 8 times

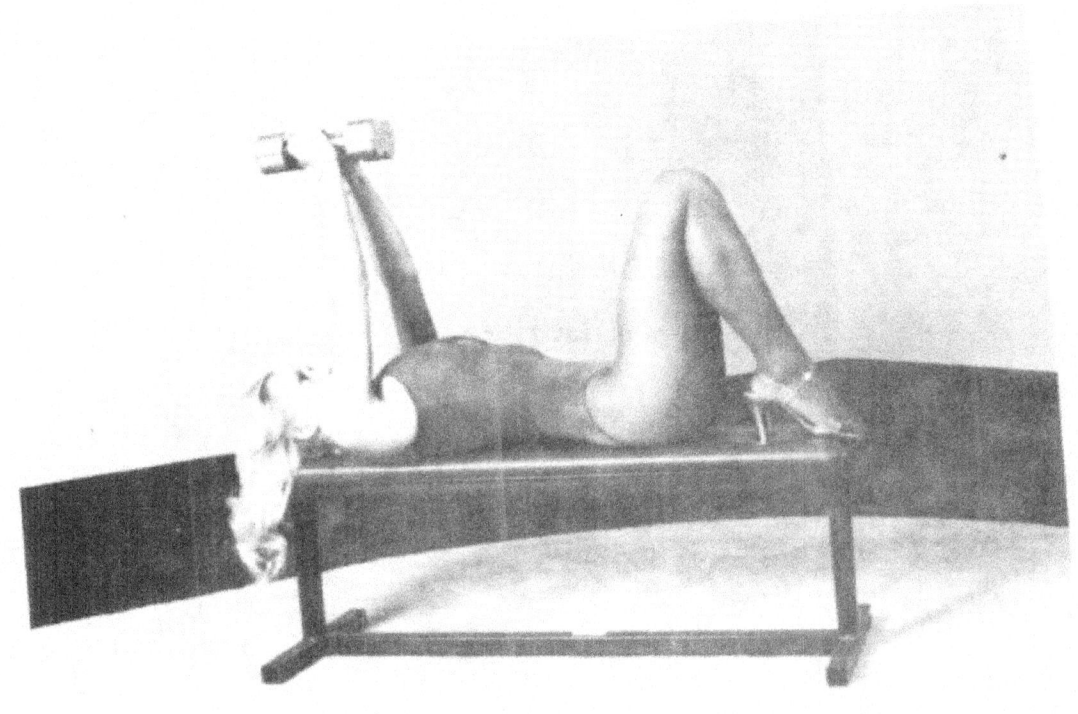

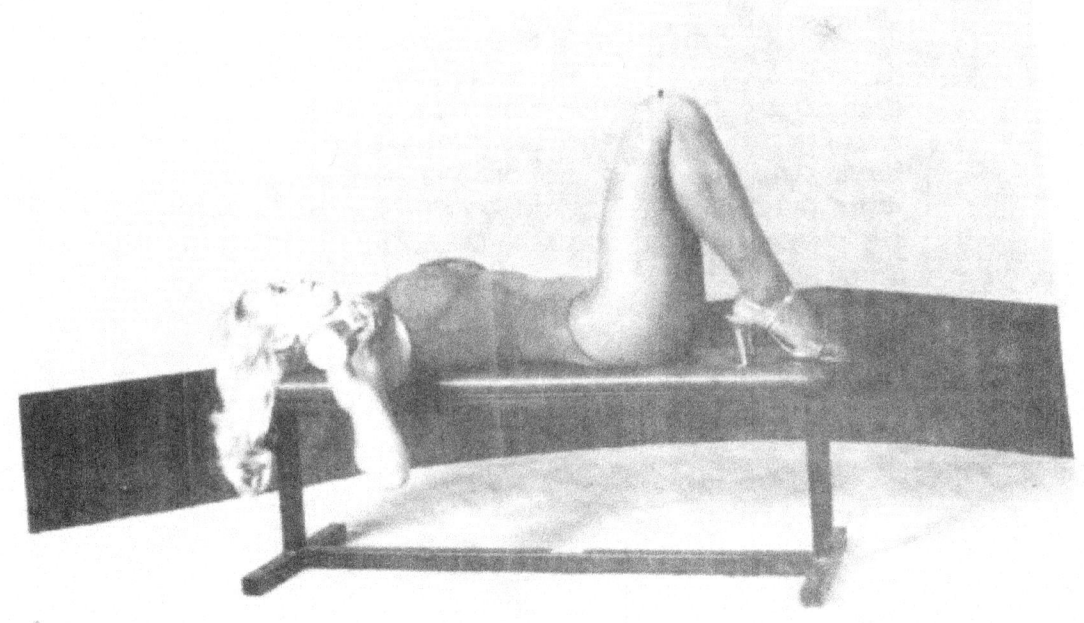

EXERCISE NUMBER **23:**   BUTTERFLIES

EQUIPMENT NEEDED: Incline board or lawn
chair, two dumbell

DIRECTONS:
   Sit on an incline board with knees bent and feet on the floor,
holding a pair of dumbells directly above the head. Begin to move
the weights around your body to the sides in a vary large circle---
holding them at arm's length.Circle until the weights come together
at the bottom of the circle, just above the pelvis.
   Bend the arms, and return the weights to the original position.
Be sure the weights do not drop too low at the sides and be sure to
bring them together at the bottom before begnning again. The
circles are slow, methodical movements, not wild flailings of the
arms.
   Repeat 8 times.

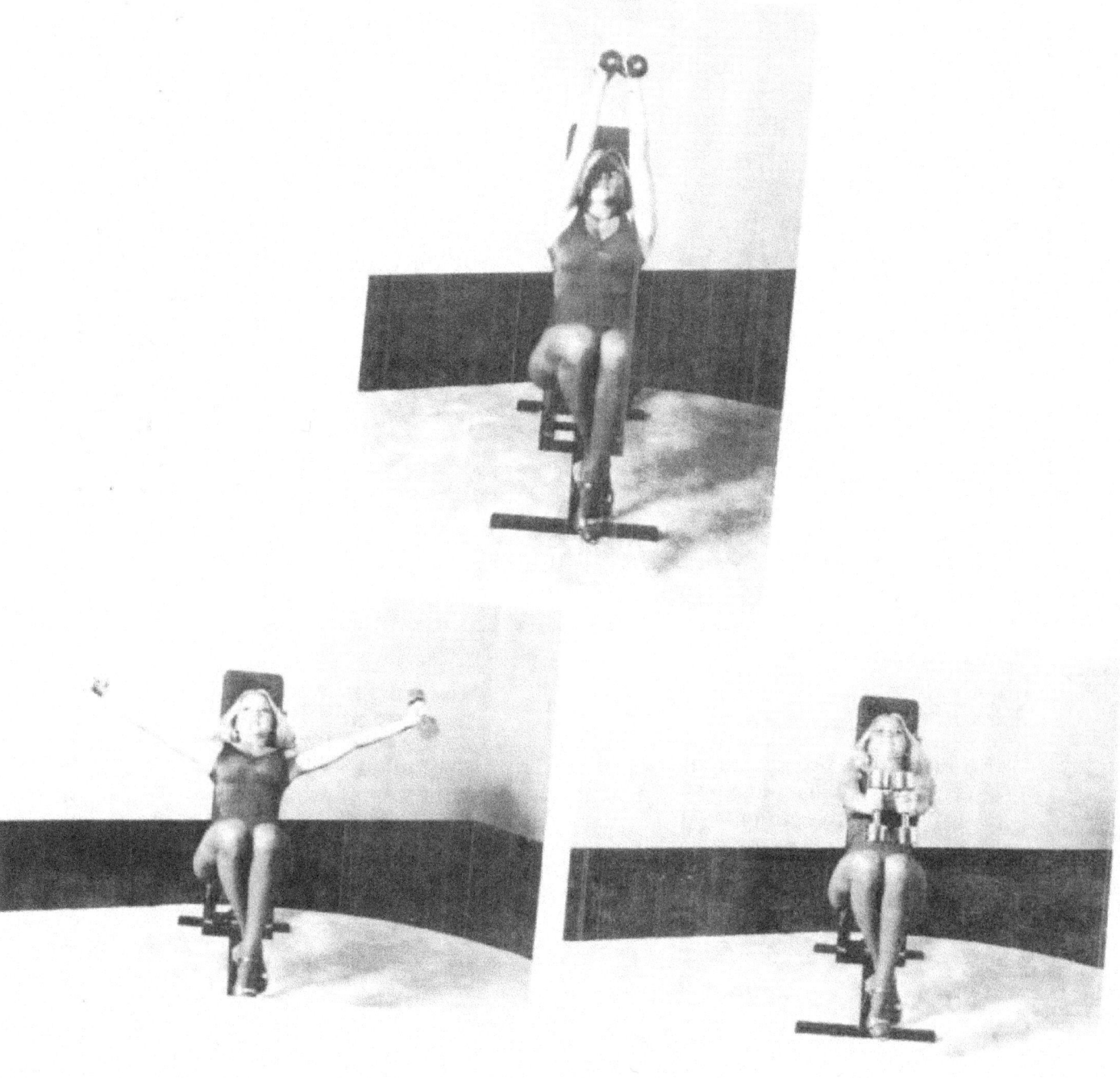

EXERCISE NUMBER 24   PECTORAL PUSH

EQUIPMENT NEEDED: BUTTERFLY MACHINE

DIRECTIONS:
     This exercise works like doing flys, but is more effective because the machine isolates the muscles. Sit in the machine with the arms extended back so that they grab the handles on the machine. Take a deep breath and begin to push the arms together so that the elbows touch in front of the body.
     Hold this position a few seconds concentrating on the squeezing of the chest muscles. Slowly let the weights return to the original position.
     Repeat 8 to 15 times.

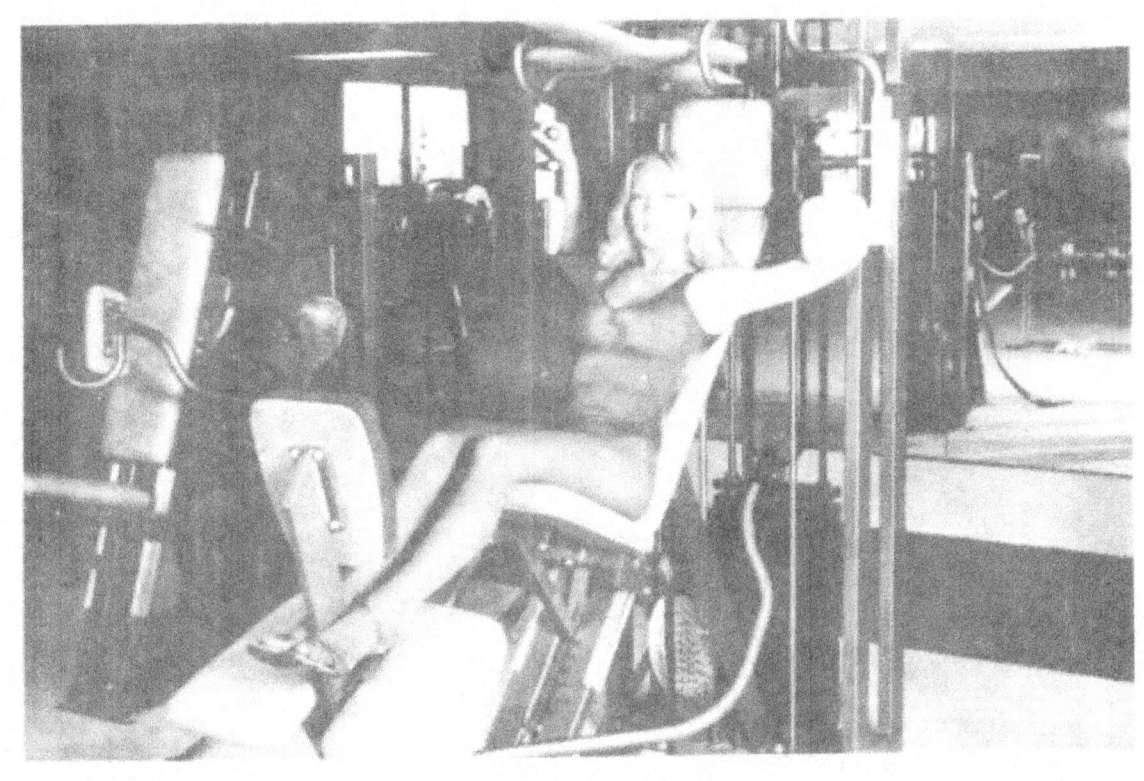

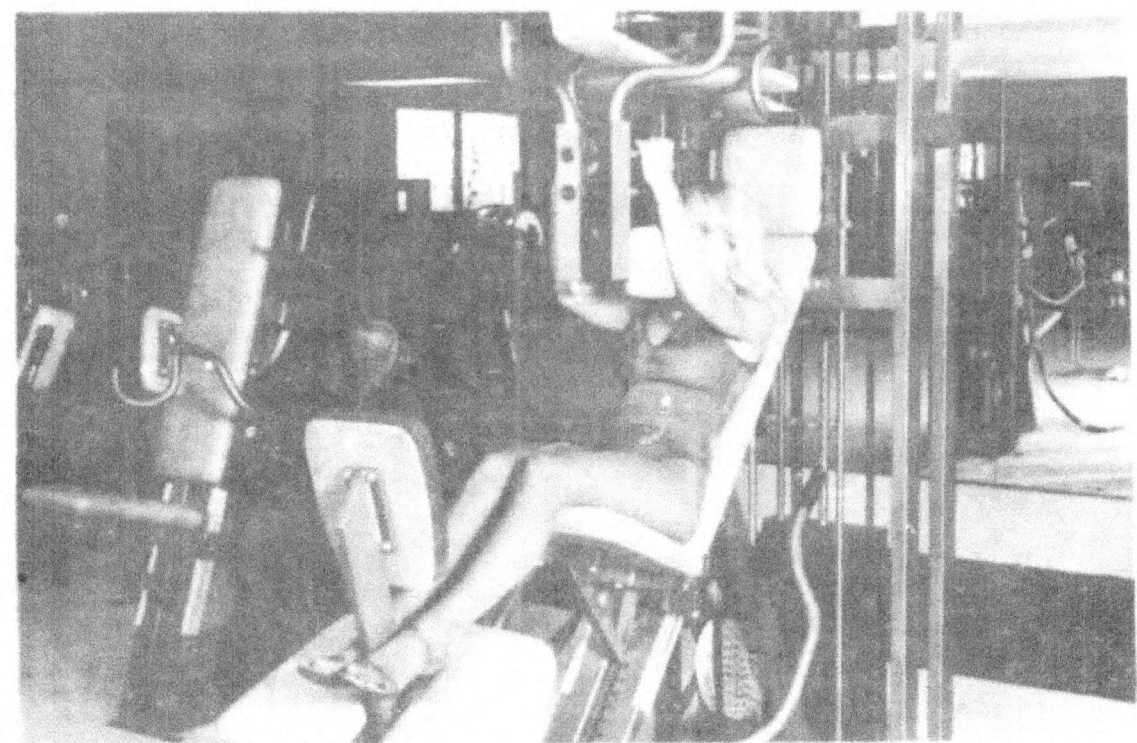

EXERCISE NUMBER 25:   REVERSE FLYS

EQUIPMENT NEEDED: BUTTERFLY MACHINE

DIRECTIONS:
    Sit in the machine facing backwards, towards the weights. Have a partner hand you the resistance arms, and place the elbows firmly against the pads.
    Take a deep breath and begin to push on the pads towards the back of your body. Push as far back as you can go. Hold this full extension a few seconds, then slowly return to the starting position.
    Repeat this exercise 8 to 15 times.

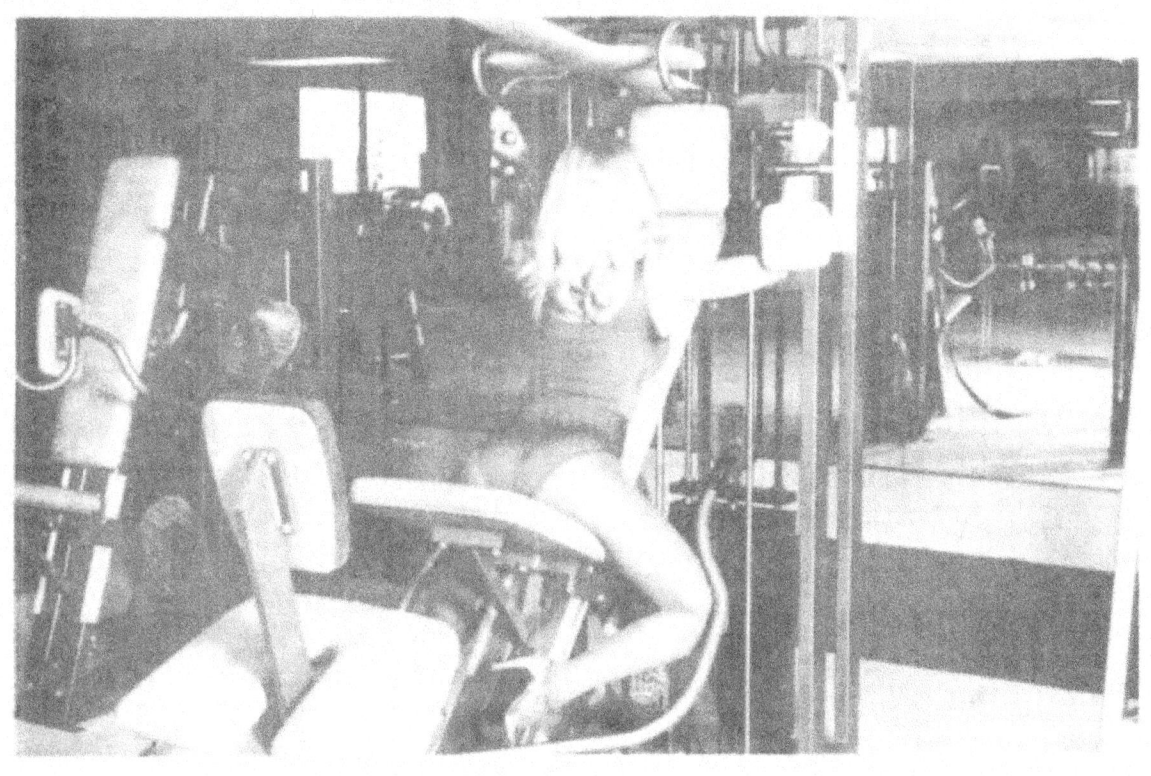

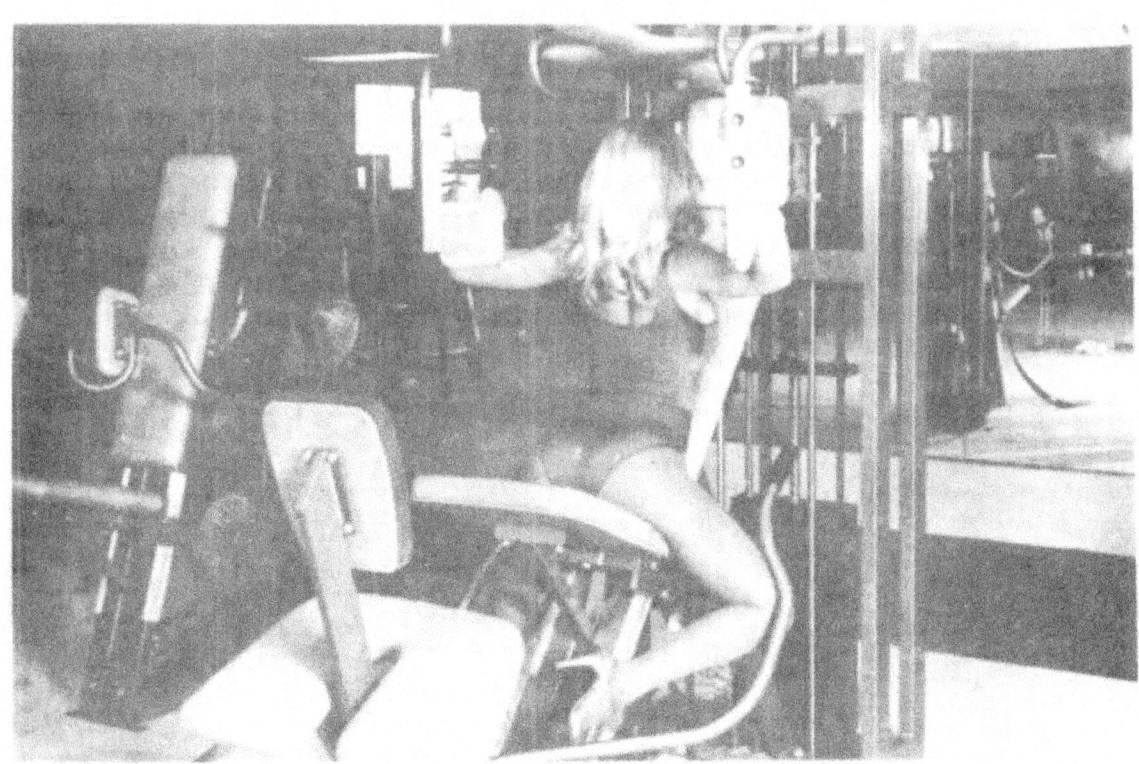

EXERCISE NUMBER 26: INCLINE FLYS

EQUIPMENT NEEDED: Dumbells, incline bench or slanted chair

DIRECTIONS:
Sit on the incline bench holding a pair of light (5 to 10 pound) dumbells extended over the head at arms length. Keep the palms facing away from the body. Slowly lower the weights in a slight arch to each side until the arms can go no further without dropping the weights. As strength grows, the stretch widens, thus increasing the effectiveness of the exercise.

Hold this full extension for four seconds, then squeezing the chest muscles together, lift the weights back to the starting position.

Repeat this exercise 8 to 15 times.

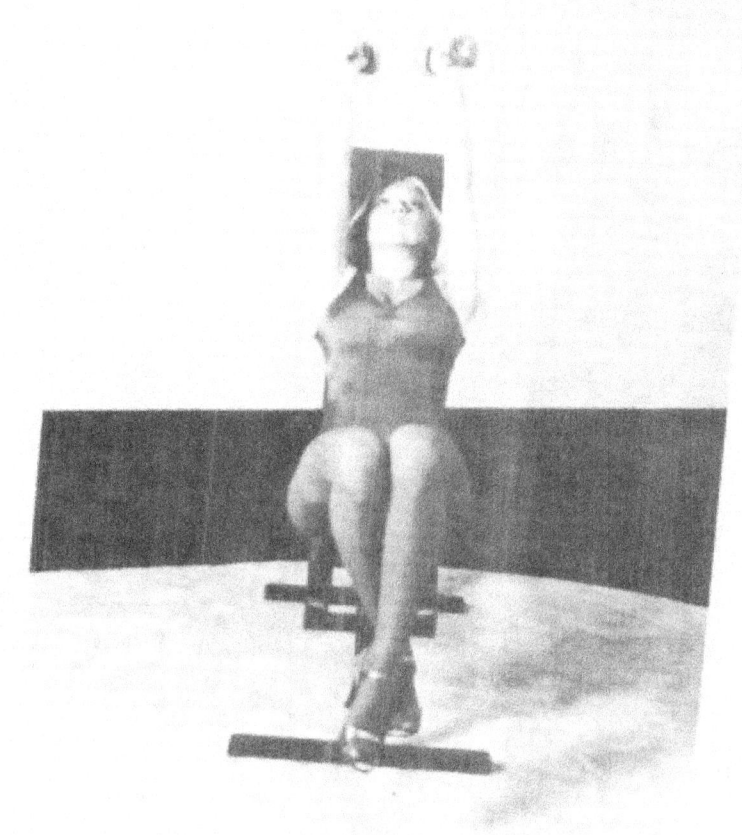

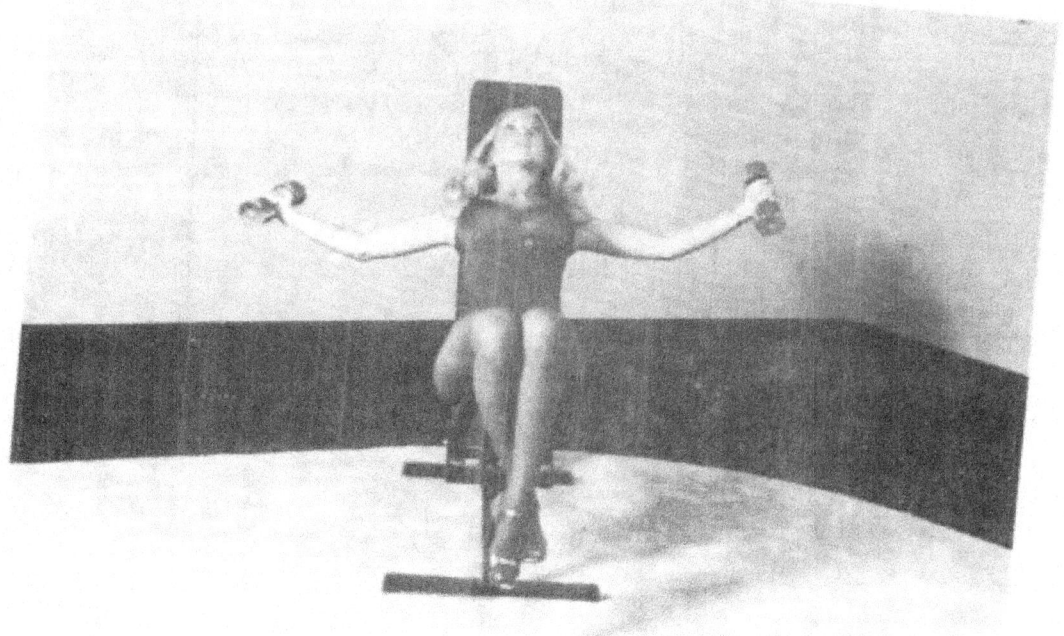

EXERCISE NUMBER 27:   DIPS BETWEEN CHAIRS

EQUIPMENT NEEDED: Two benches, or two chairs
with non skid surfaces

DIRECTIONS:
   If you have too much difficulty doing regular dips you can try this
exercise, it is quite effective and will help to develop the tops of the
busts.
   Secure two chairs or benches so that they do not slide. Keeping
the feet on the floor hold yourself supported by your arms in a straight
angle between the two chairs. Slowly lower yourself down until your
chest is well below your palms.
   Hold this full stretch for a few seconds, then push yourself back
up to the original position. Repeat this 8 to 15 times.

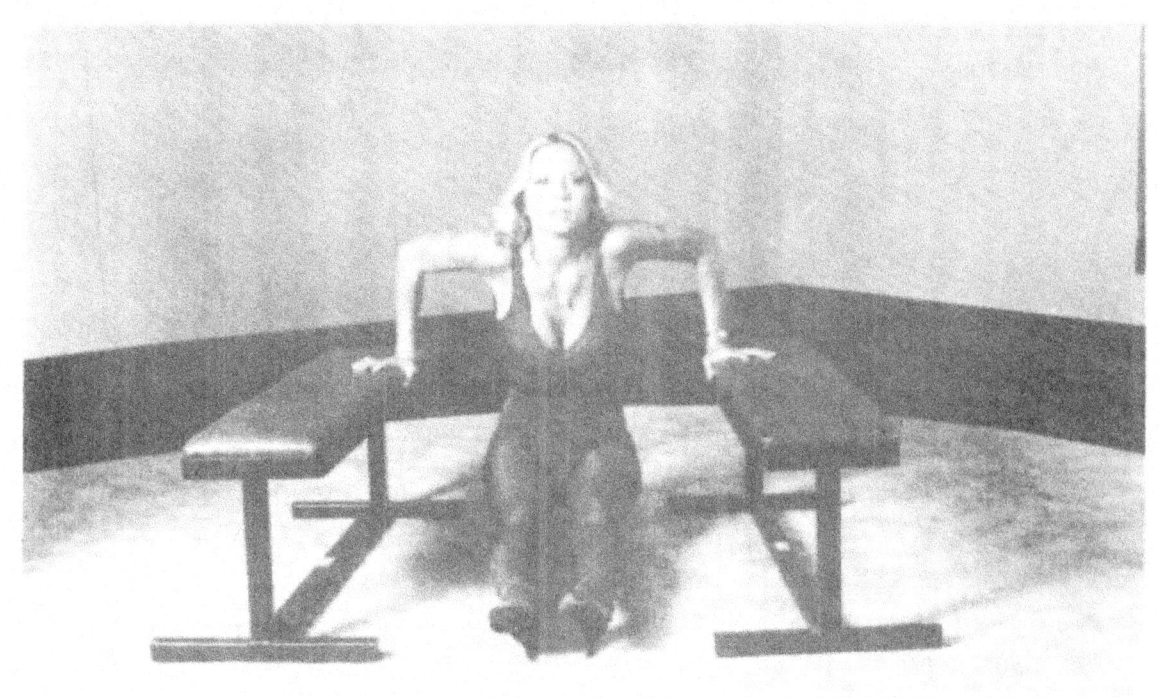

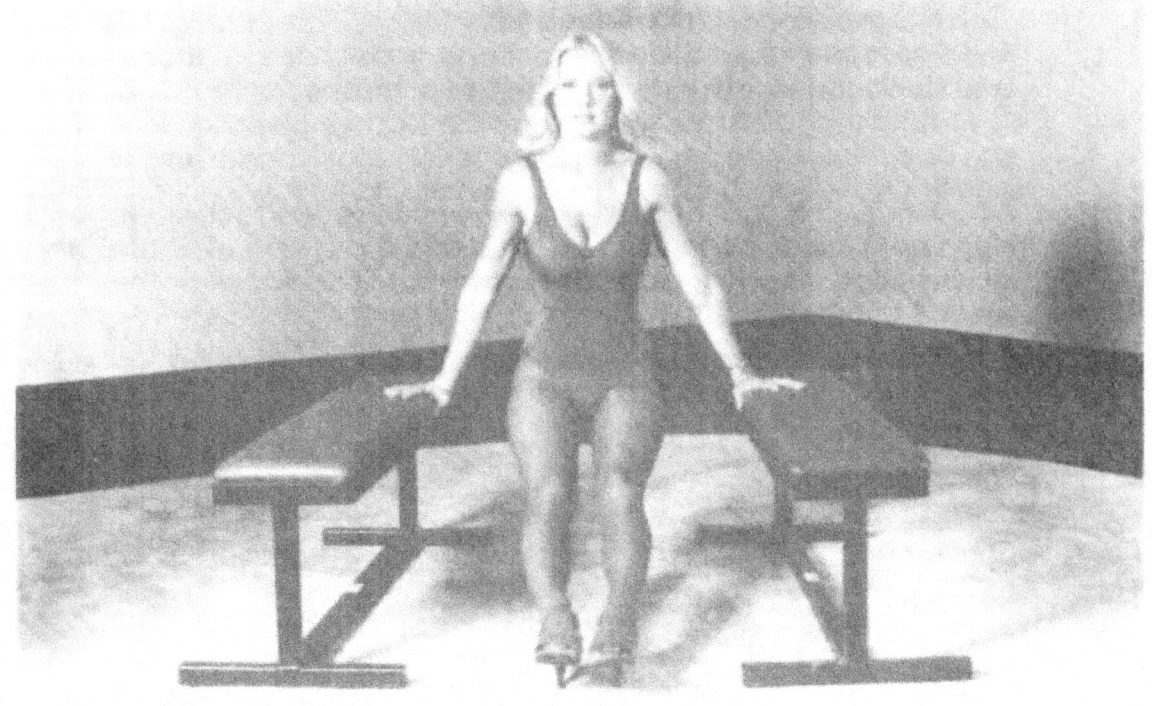

EXERCISE NUMBER 28:   DIPS

EQUIPMENT NEEDED: dipping bar, or two chairs secured on the floor so that they do not slip, and high enough for your body to be suspended in the air.

DIRECTIONS:

Hold your body suspended off the ground. Take a deep breath and slowly lower your body down between the bars until your chest is at the same height as your palms, or slightly lower.

Hold this full stretch for four seconds, then blow out your air, and begin to lift your body back up to the original starting position.

Although this exercise is strenous it is very effective and will do much to develop your bust if done properly. If you can not do the dip with all your body weight, you may begin with doing chair dips and work your way up to the regular dips.

Do as many dips as possible, being sure to use good form.

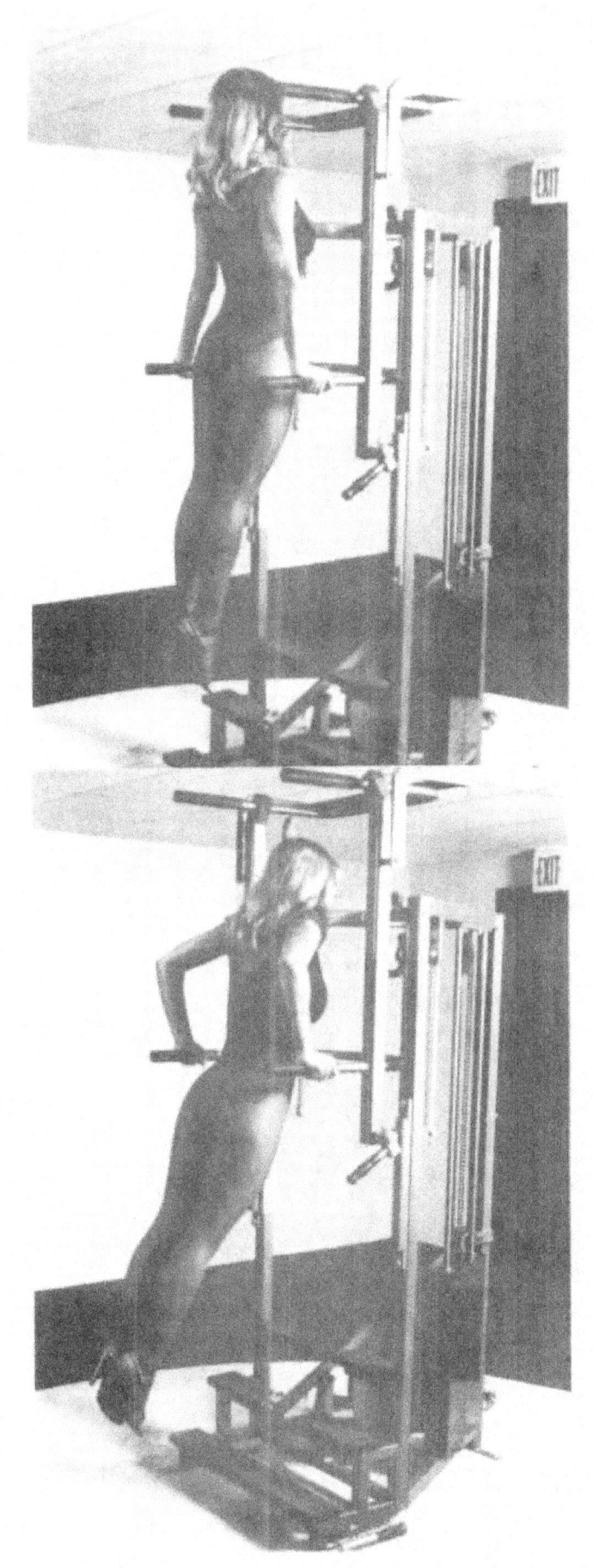

EXERCISE NUMBER 29:   INVERTED PUSH UP

EQUIPMENT NEEDED: NONE

DIRECTIONS:
    Lie on your back with your elbows down by your sides. Take a
deep breath and using ther strength of your elbows and bust
muscles, begin to lift yourself off the ground until your body weight
is fully supported by the elbows.
    Hold this full extension a few seconds, then slowly let yourself
back down, concentrating on the muscles of the bust.
    Repeat 8 to 15 times.

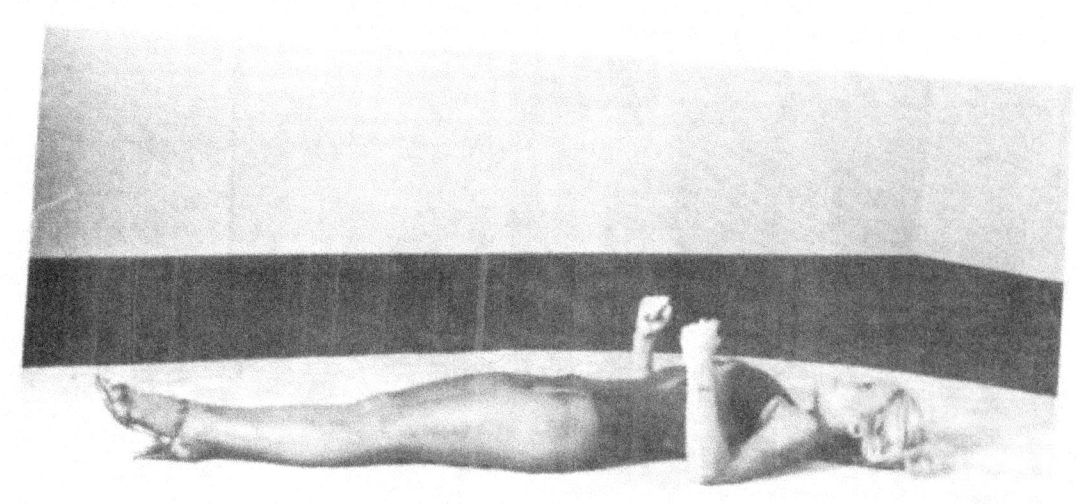

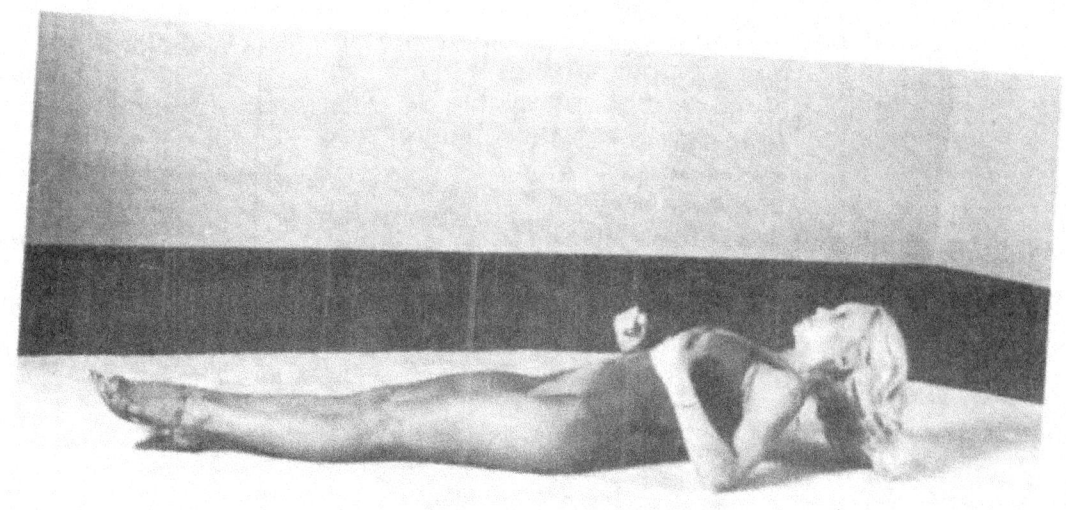

EXERCISE NUMBER 30:   ISOMETRIC SQUEEZE

EQUIPMENT NEEDED: NONE

DIRECTIONS:
Stand with the feet about shoulder width apart and the back straight. Reach across your bust with the right arm and grab your left elbow with the right hand. Begin to pull on the left elbow and begin to concentrate on tightening the muscles of the chest,until you can actually feel the chest muscles tighten.

Hold this full tightening for 8 seconds, then relax and repeat the exercise 4 more times.

This exercise is easy to do, and you can really feel it working the muscles of the chest, causing the bust to grow.

Repeat this exercise 4 to 8 times.

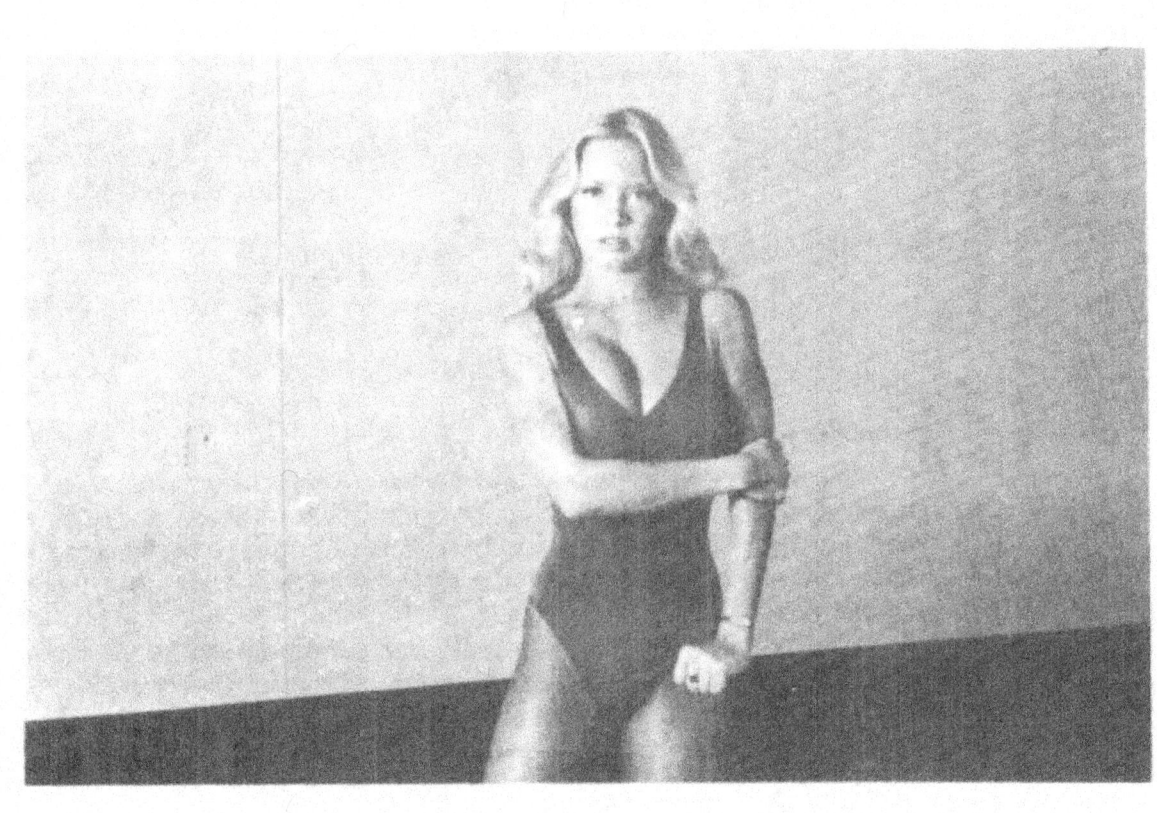

EXERCISE NUMBER 31:   RESISTANCE BUTTERFLY
                    (with partner)

EQUIPMENT NEEDED: A partner

DIRECTIONS:
    Stand directly in front of the partner with your elbows in front of
your chest. Let your partner grasp your elbows with his hands and hold
them tightly. Now take a deep breath and begin to try to open your
elbows up as he tries to resist your doing so. Try as hard as you can for
at least 8 seconds.
    This exercise is isometric and isotonic in that it works the muscles
using another muscle as a resistor and also works the muscles using
another persons muscles as a resistance.
    Repeat this exercise 4 times.

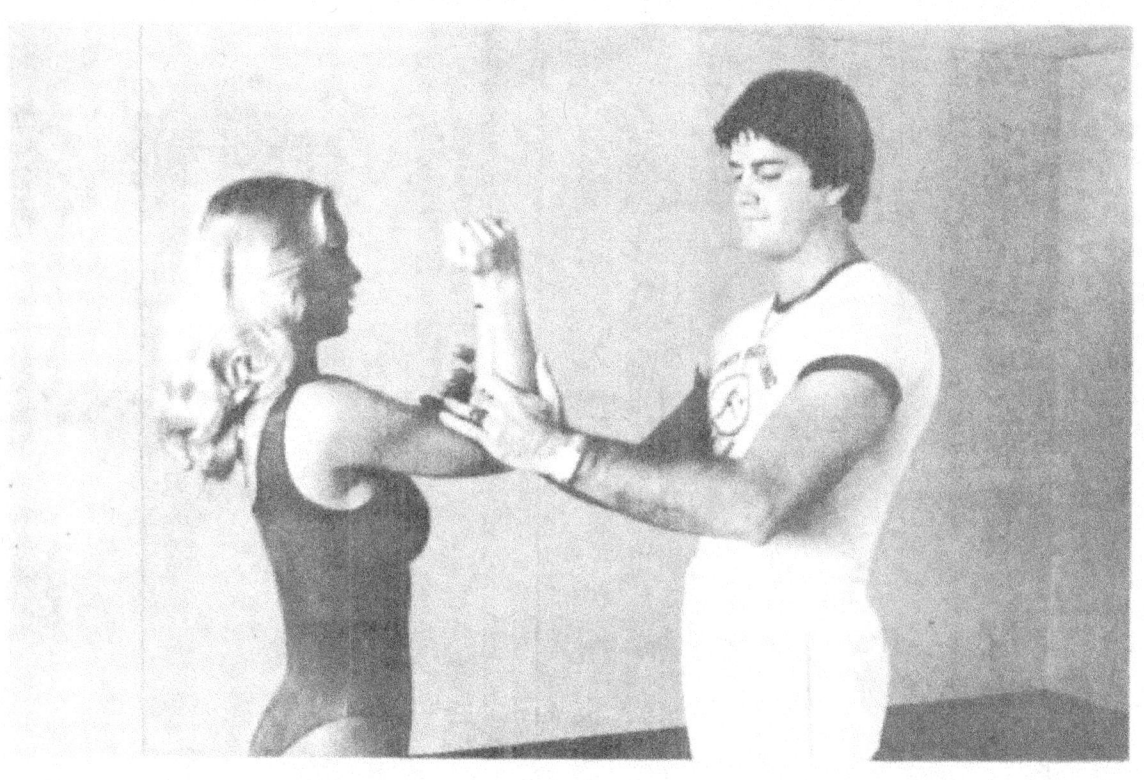

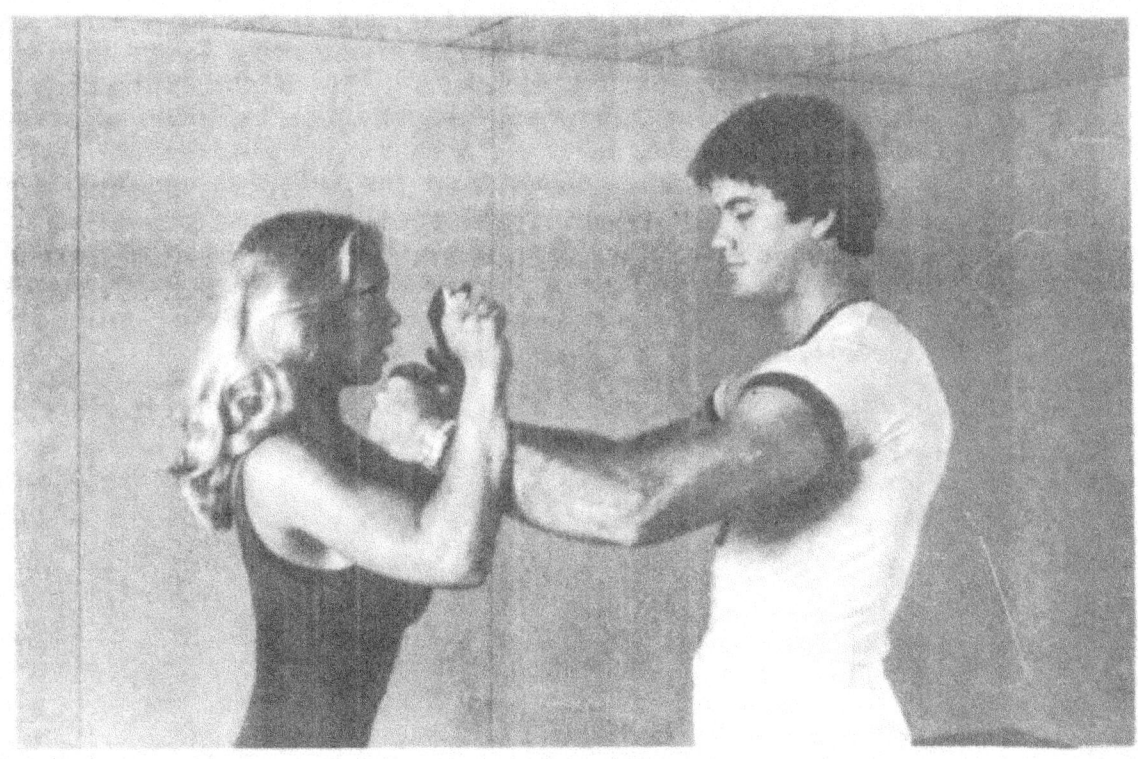

EXERCISE NUMBER 32:   RESISTANCE FLYS (with partner)

EQUIPMENT NEEDED: a partner

DIRECTIONS:

Have the partner stand behind you and grasp your arms as you hold them fully extended to the sides of your body. Take a deep breath and begin to try to bring the arms together in front of the body. The partner should let you move very slightly, resisting all the way to really work your muscles.

When your arms touch in front , the partner should stop resisting and let you return your arms to the back. Note: your partner will not be able to follow your arms all the way to the front, but it is only necessary for him to follow you as you first begin your movement. That is where the most muscle resistance is happening and the most growth will take place.

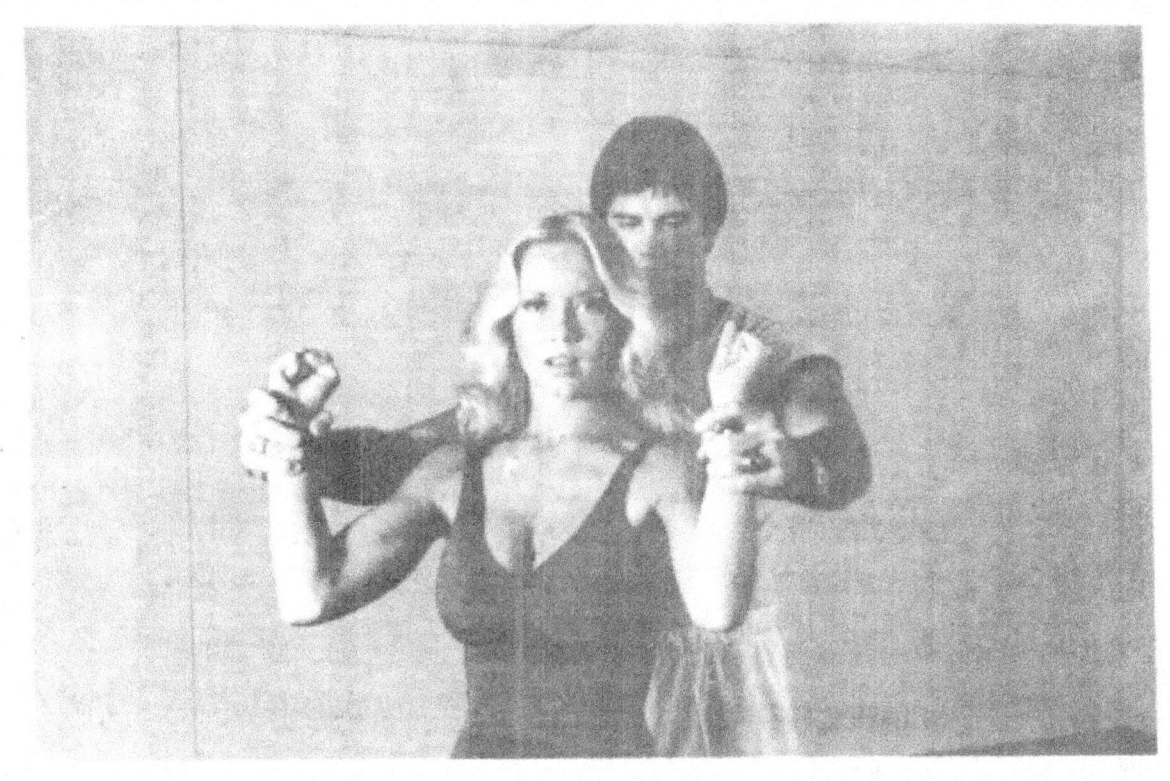

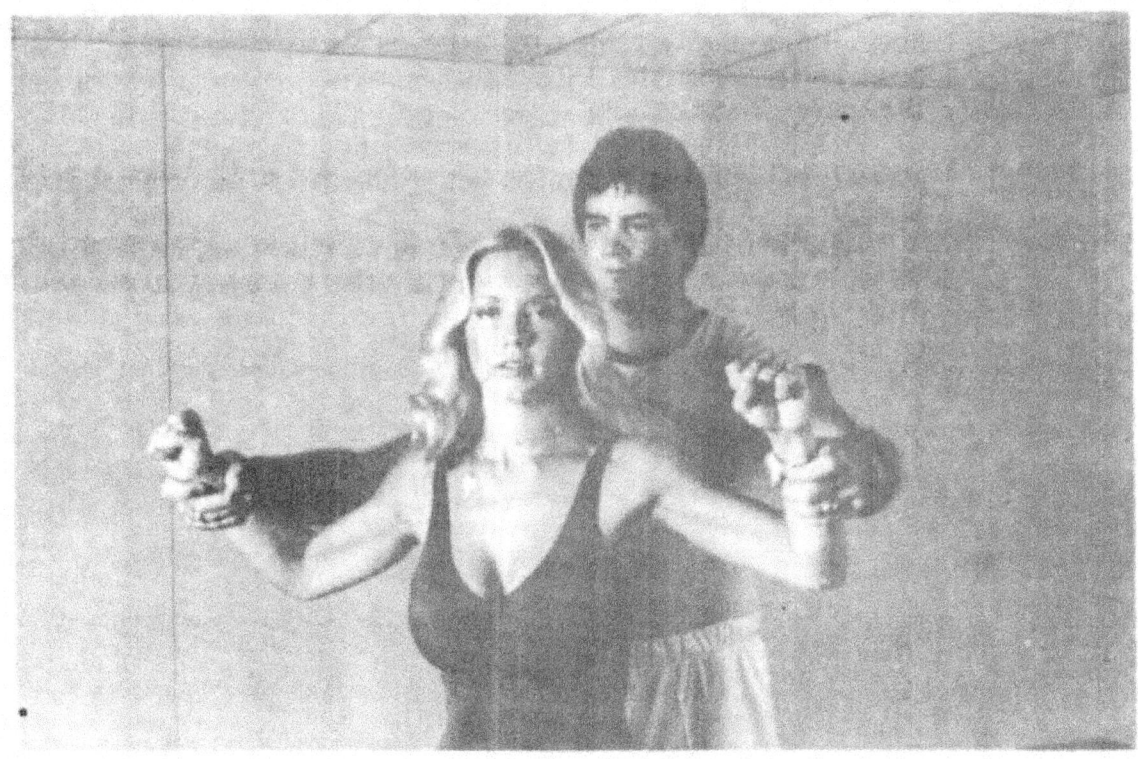

EXERCISE NUMBER 33:   PULLOVERS

EQUIPMENT NEEDED: Dumbells, flat bench or two stools.

DIRECTIONS:

Lie flat on your back on the bench with a dumbell suspended over your chest. Hold the dumbell in your hands with the palms facing towards the ceiling. Take a deep breath and slowly begin to lower the dumbell down over the top of your head and towards the floor. Try to stretch the arms back as far as they can go over the head and towards the floor. Be carefull not to bend the arms or lift the back off the bench.

Hold this full extension a few seconds, then blow out all of your air as you begin to return the weight back to the original starting position.

You should use a weight that is comfortable, usually around 15 to 25 pounds is enough. As your strength grows you may want to increase the poundage.

Do this exercise 8 to 15 times.

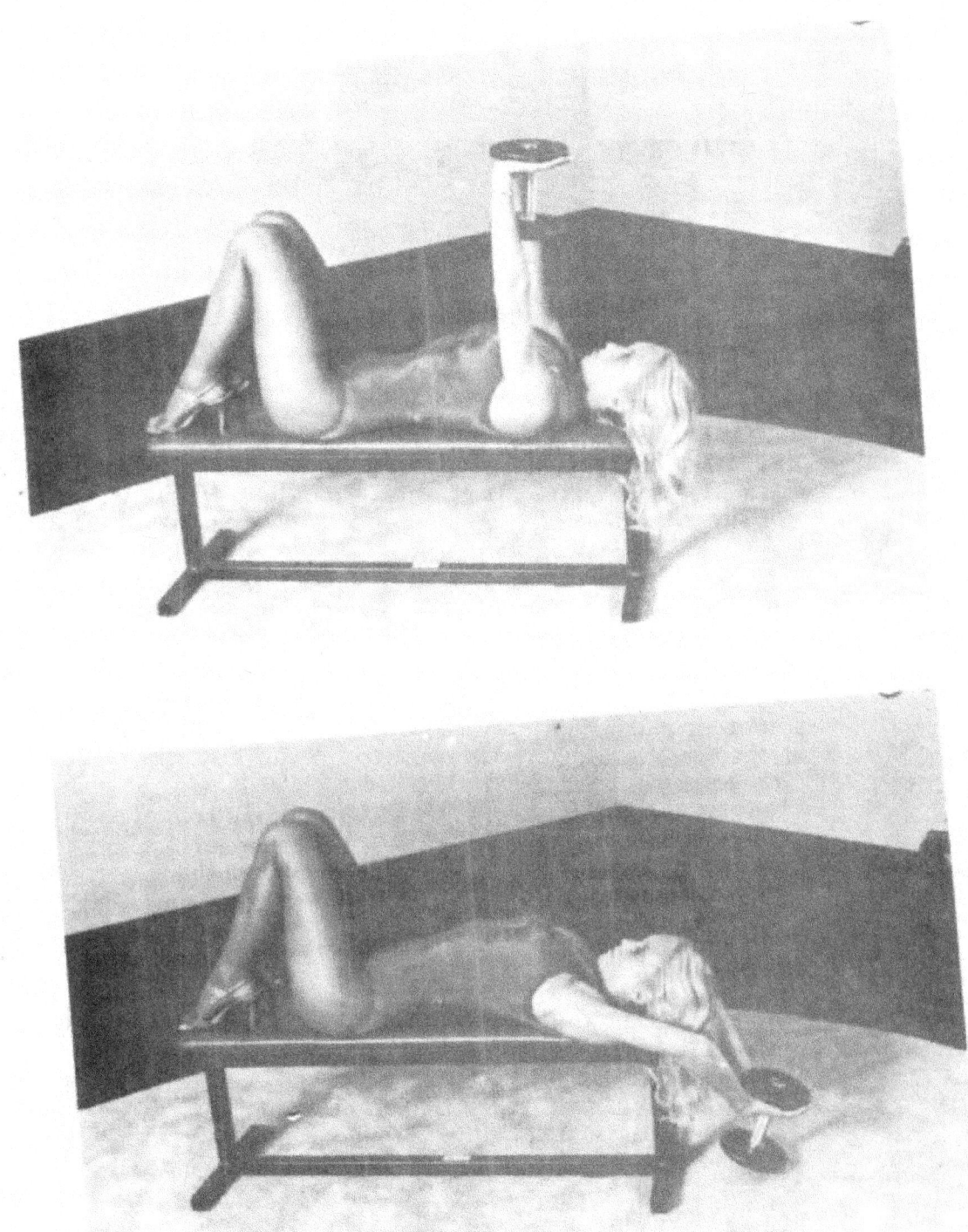

HYPNOTISM: SUBCONCIOUS CONDITIONING

Hypnotism is helpful in aiding concentration, thereby increasing the results form any exercise program. It can help to increase the supply of blood to the chest area, bringing more protein and enzymes which can aid bust growth.

Many psychiatists, medical doctors, and state licensed hypnotism clinics offer hypnosis help, though many people prefer to practice self-hyponosis or auto-suggestion. Meditation, and the "trance state" associated with deep meditation are forms of self-hypnosis.

Before submitting to hypnosis by anyother person, check their references throughly. Your local medical society, Better Business Bureau and Chamber of Commerce are good sources of information.

The directions given here for self-hypnosis are completely safe--there is nothing to worry about. The worst thing that could happen in the unlikely event of too much auto-suggestion is a relaxing, if unexpected, nap.

Take a few deep breaths and gently close your eyes. Imagine you are walking up some steps to the second floor of a house where feelings are very comfortable and the surroundings are familiar. With each step taken your drowsiness and sleepy feeling are increasing. Making it to the top without going to sleep begins to seem impossible.

Imagine that after each step, you pause to take a breath, and after each breath and step drowsiness increases. With only 10 steps to go, you should feel very, very sleepy, with arms and legs so heavy they can barely be moved.

Take the last few steps, and let yourself feel as if you are going to sleep. By the last step, the feeling should resemble a very deep sleep. At this stage your mind should seem to be floating and the feelings should be very relaxed and happy. Only then is it possible to suggest that desirable things happen. It is important to remember that hypnotism, whether done by a professional or self-induced, can only suggest certain things the mind wishes to happen. Hypnotism cannot suggest or cause any actions that the mind finds objectionable.

Say to yourself "I want my bust to grow and grow and I will do all the exercises exactly right every day until I get the results I want. I will not miss a day or skip an exercise. I will look forward to doing the exercises because I want my bust to grow and I will enjoy working to make it grow."

Again and again repeat the instructions, "I will do all my exercises and not skip or cheat and my bust will grow and grow until it is as large and as firm as I want it to be." If a specific target goal has been set, such as an increase of three inches, substitute that goal where appropriate in the instructions.

After all the instructions have been relayed to the sub-concious, begin to think of waking up. Slowly counting to 10 become more and more awake until a feeling of alert good health is reached by the final number.

Some people find that recording a message in their own voice works better than simply imagining the instructions. Follow the same relaxation techniques, substituting the tape for the silent mental commands outlined above.

Repeat this hypnosis exercise daily until all goals for the program are reached.

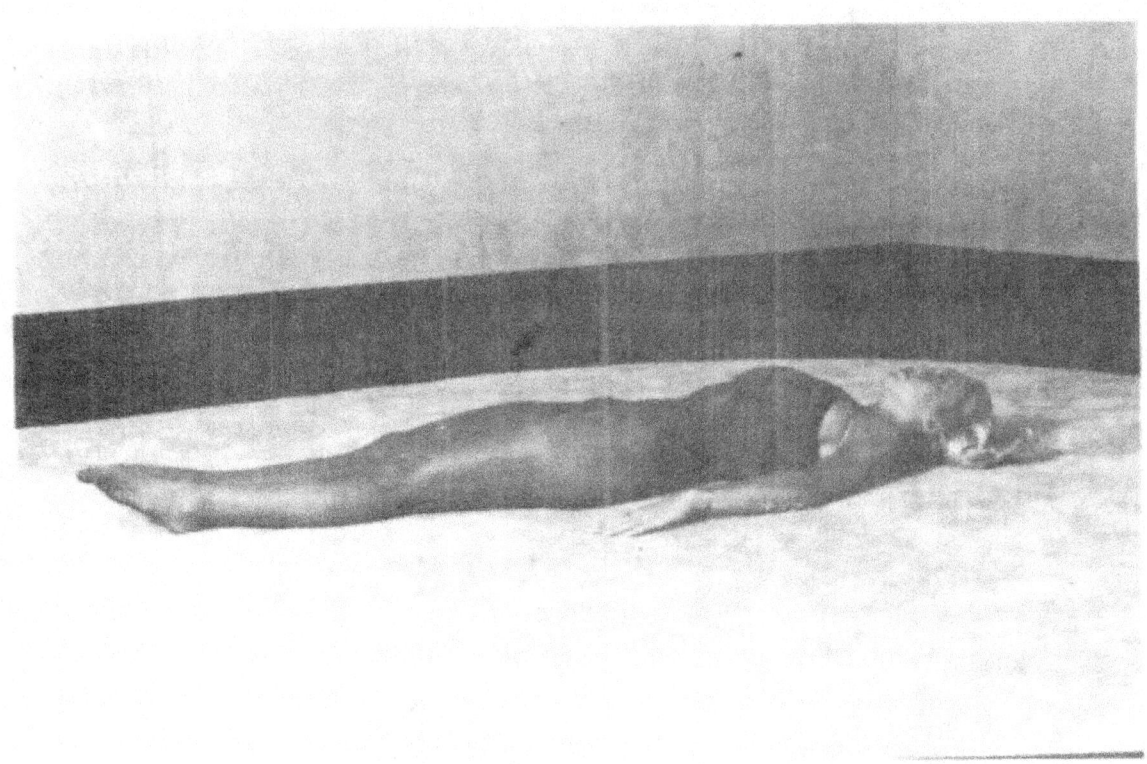

MEDITATION: MIND OVER MUSCLE

Many professionals believe that meditation can be very useful in developing the chest by using the power of the mind to increase the blood supply to the bust. Increased blood flow brings more protein and enzymes into the chest area, which aids development and growth.

To try a simple mediation, sit on the floor on a cushion if desired, in the half-lotus position, one leg on top of the other (Indian style).

Keep the back straight and the eyes slightly or fully closed. Take a few deep breaths and relax yourself more and more with each breath. Concentrating only on the breathings begin to follow each breath in and out of your body.

Imagine the breath as a silver thread and follow it through the body as you breath. Begin to follow it through the nose, and down the throat into the lungs, then throughout the body. Follow each breath in and out of the body. Relax, and try not to be disturbed by any other thoughts...just follow the silver thread.

After a few minutes of the exercise, the mind should become very relaxed and control will become easier. Begin to concentrate the mind on building the bust, imagining that the heart is beating very hard. Follow in the mind the blood as it leaves the heart and flows through the body. Because you want your bust to grow, concentrate especially on the blood being drawn to the chest and filling the chest with blood and power. Imagine that the bust is growing with every breath and is getting stronger and stronger with each beat of the heart. Imagine the bust growing and getting stronger as you breathe in and out.

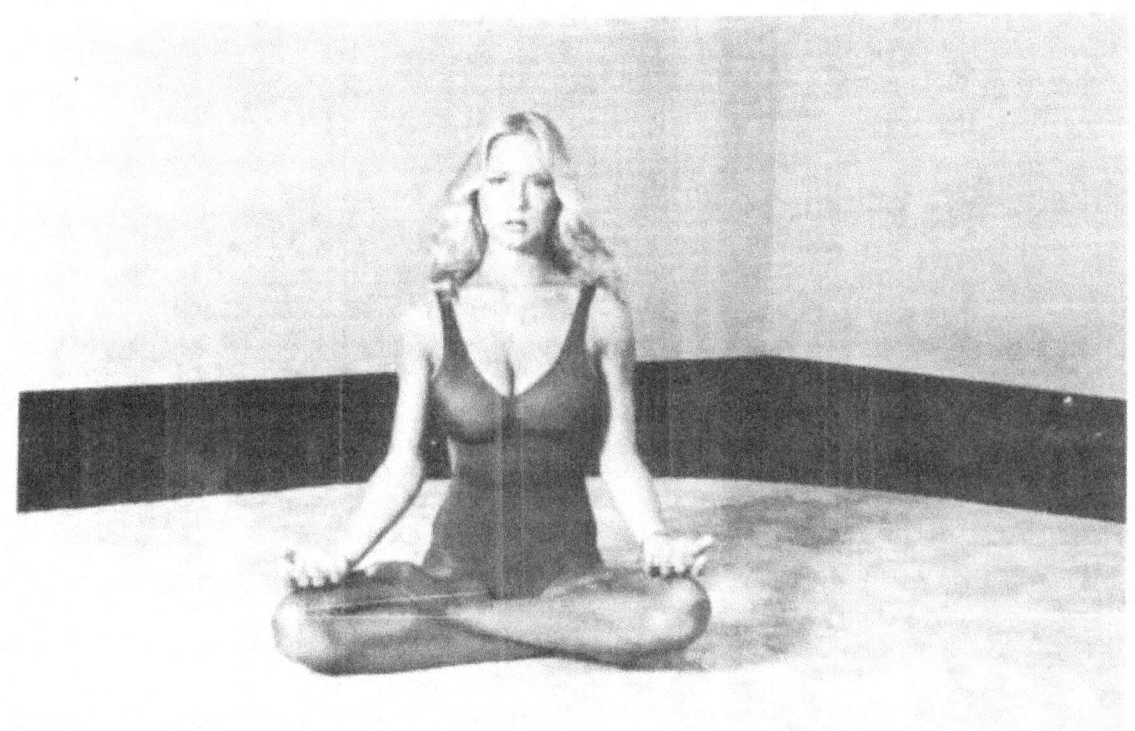

Concentrate the mind on the fact that more blood is coming to the chest with each breath and this blood is causing the chest to grow. Picture in the mind's eye the chest growing and growing. Do this about 5 to 15 minutes, or as long as it is possible to concentrate only on the blood causing the chest to grow.

If the mind starts to wander too much, get up and stop the meditation, it does no good unless concentration is complete. As concentration ends, take a few deep breaths and repeat to yourself "I feel wonderful, alive, and beautiful". Do this exercise daily.

ENZYMES: BUILDING BLOCKS AND CATALYSTS FOR GROWTH

Enzymes are a group of proteins that function as catalysts in bio-chemical reactions. In other words, they enable the body to exhange one vital commodity for another, such as food for energy, or changing protein into muscle. They act as go betweens and regulate the amount of energy that is required for chemical reactions to take place rapidly.

One of the most often used is a substance called Adenosine Triphosphate (ATP) which serves as a carrier of reactions between cells that supply energy and those that use it. ATP serves various functions in this role, such as transportation of materials into cells, conducting nerve signals throughout the body, cell division and regulations, synthesis of protein, muscle construction and regula-tion of body temperature.

While it is generally assumed that an adequate diet supplemented by a good multi-vitamin will supply all the necessary enzymes or co-enzymes, is always a chance that not enough enzymes are available for the body to grow to its full potential. Therefore, it is important to carefully control the diet during this exercise program to assure the proper amount of protein and vitamins. I recommend that a protein supplement be considered .Enzyme formulas that supply additional enzymes are also available at health food stores. Check with your doctor to see if he feels you might have an enzyme deficiency.

Enzymes are necessary for growth of new tissue and the development of the bust. No additional growth will take place due only to an enzyme activity. Exercise is also required. Enzyme creams, pills or capsules will merely help normal cell growth for replacement of dying cells, which occur during normal life functions. The body MUST be exercising and using its muscles very hard in order for them to grow and get stronger.

Ads claiming "remarkable enzyme cream for bust growth" should be investigated throughly, as there is no scientific evidence that proves bust growth can be achieved without exercise, or just with the use of a enzyme cream.

SURGERY: the FINAL SOLUTION.

Our last and final discussion of a technique for the development of the bust is the "final solution", surgery. Surgery is of course the only solution that requires no exercise, no diet control, no meditation, and even no long wait. It only requires money and a competant doctor.

There are various forms of surgery that are currently being used to develop the bust. The two most common are implants and silicone. Both have there advantages and both have there drawbacks. I suggest that if you are interested in finding out more about either of these techniques you consult a physican who practices these techniques.

From my research I have found out that most operations take a few hours to preform and cost a few thousand dollars. The breast can be enlarged to almost any desired size, within reason, and few side effects are noted. But if there is a complication it is usually a serious one. Like the collaspe of a breast, or the development of a extremly hard an insensitive breast.

If you follow the program outlined in my book you will not require surgery because the program really works, and will really develop your bust size. Do the exercises described, take your vitamins and watch your diet. Stick with your program and in about three months you will see a larger and firmer bust. Most women who have followed my program report a cup size difference in as little as three months. You should be able to have the size and firmness you want in a few short months and be able to keep it for the rest of your life by maintaining a sensible exercise and diet program.

GLOSSARY

BARBELLS: Free weights on a single bar. Barbells require the use of both hands simultaneously.

BREAST: The soft, protruding mannary gland. Used for milk storage during pegnancy.

BUST: The area of the chest surrounding the breasts, particularly the pectoral muscles.

DECLINES: A board or bench which declines at approximately a 35 degree angle. When lying on it, the subjects head is down and the feet are elevated. It is used to work the lower chest muscles.

DUMBELLS: Free weights on a small bar, held in each hand separately. The bars may be used simultaneously or exercised one arm at a time.

ENZYME: A group of proteins used in the metabolism of food. Enzymnes serve as catalysts in metabolism and are necessary for growth.

EXTENSION: The point where maximun stretch is reached. The point at which the arms or weights can go no farther away from the body.

INCLINES: A board or bench which is inclined at about a 35 degree angle. When using an incline board the subjects head is up and their feet are down. It is used to work the top portion of your pectoral muscles.

ISOMETRIC: Muscles working against muscles. This exercise technique requires no weights or machines, for resistance is achieved by the opposition of your muscles.

MEDITATION: Concentration of ones mind on one specific thought or idea to such an extent that no other thoughts distract or distrub your concentration.

PECTORAL: The large muscle that composes the area around the breast. This muscle is what can be built, firmed and toned by exercise.

PROTEIN: A group of 22 amino acids, necessary for growth and life. Proteins compose over 80% of muscle mass.

REPETITIONS: The amount of times you perform a particular exercise. A set is composed of a group of repetitions.

SET: A group of repetitions of a certain exercise. All sets should be done together for the same muscle group.

SPRINGS: An exercise device that employs the use of springs as a form of resisance.

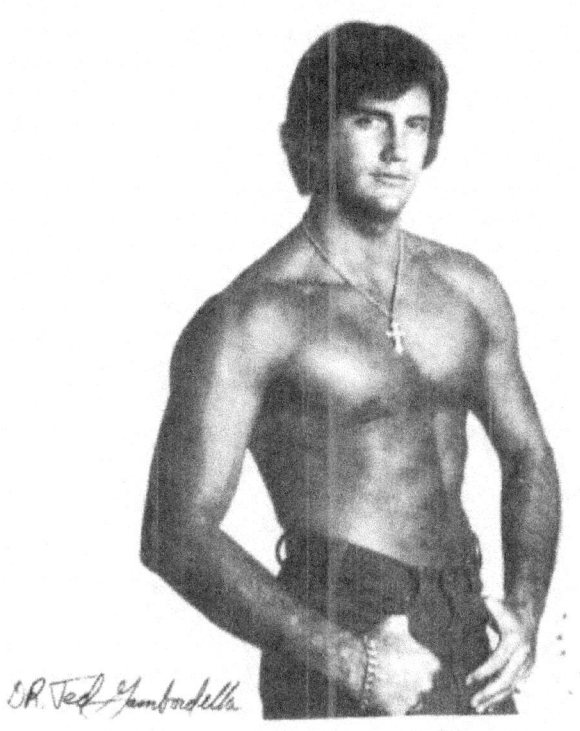

Dr. Ted Gambordella

ABOUT THE AUTHOR

Ted Gambordella has been active in the physical fitness field for over 10 years and has served as manager and supervisor of various health spas. He is a former director of the Sports Medicine Clinic of Dallas.

He holds Bachelor's and Master's Degrees from Louisiana State University in guidance and counseling and physical education, and holds a non-academic Martial Arts Doctorate from the University of the Orient. He is a Black Belt martial arts expert, and the U.S. Senior Karate Champion 1980, who lifts weights, jogs and works out daily to keep his body fit.

He is the author of the nationally recognized injury prevention program "END OF INJURY", which has been endorsed by top colleges and universities across the country, including the University of Oklahoma, the University of Texas, Rice, L.S.U., and professional basketball and soccer.

His other works include:
HOW TO DEVELOP A PERFECT BODY IN 30 MINUTES A DAY.
SEVEN DAYS TO SELF DEFENSE.
THE COMPLETE BOOK OF WEAPONS.
HOW TO DEVELOP A PERFECT WAISTLINE
29 WAYS TO PREVENT BALDNESS
SELF DEFENSE FOR CHILDREN
THE MARVELOUS MENTAL DIET.

Gambordella has worked with many of the top universities and professional teams in the U.S. and has a regular television program on exercise on Channel 11 in Dallas. He also writes several columns for newspapers on health and fitness and is a much sought after counsultant on the subjects of health, fitness and